Also by Verena Tschudin:

Counselling Skills for Nurses, 4th edition (Baillière Tindall, London)

Ethics in Nursing, 2nd edition (Butterworth Heinemann, Oxford)

Ethics (a series of eight edited books) (Scutari Press, London)

Deciding Ethically (Baillière Tindall, London)

Counselling for Loss and Bereavement (Baillière Tindall, London)

Managing Yourself (Macmillan Press, Basingstoke)

Nursing the Patient with Cancer (ed.) (Prentice Hall, Hemel Hempstead)

Nurses Matter

Reclaiming our professional identity

by

Verena Tschudin

MACMILLAN

First published 1999 by
MACMILLAN PRESS LTD
Houndmills, Basingstoke, Hampshire RG21 6XS
and London
Companies and representatives throughout the world

ISBN 0–333–76054–9 paperback

A catalogue record for this book is available
from the British Library.

This book is printed on paper suitable for recycling and
made from fully managed and sustained forest sources.

10 9   8   7   6   5   4   3   2   1
08 07 06 05 04 03 02 01 00 99

Editing and origination by
Aardvark Editorial, Mendham, Suffolk

Printed in Malaysia

To Michael Wilson,
in gratitude

Contents

Preface

There are any number of reasons why nurses matter, make all the difference and are indispensable. There are just as many reasons why nurses can be dispensed with and are replaceable, and why lots of people would be quite pleased not to have them around. It is not a question of persuading these people that nurses matter but of making it so obvious and natural that they cannot do anything else but believe and acknowledge that nurses are not only indispensable in today's society, but also have a vital vision, message and role. Not only does the world need to hear that message, but also nurses have to believe that they indeed have that vision, message and role, that they can make them known and that they count.

The ideas explored in this book reach both backwards and forwards. They reach backwards in that the basis of the message and vision are considered, and forwards in that possibilities of what could be achieved are envisaged. The premise that 'people matter' is more inclusive and enhancing than other ideas that have hitherto been used to give nursing an identity. 'People matter' includes everyone: those who give and those who receive. Nurses are not seen simply as professionals giving a service but as human beings relating to other human beings in personal and professional ways. This in itself is nothing new in nursing. What is new is that nursing needs a voice and an identity more urgently than ever before. People matter, what matters to them matters, and because this matters, people are enabled to be visionary, act politically and support each other and each other's visions and actions. Much of this can only happen because people – nurses and clients and patients – can see to find within themselves the creativity to say 'yes' when needed and to say 'no' when it matters.

These ideas are not in any way ground breaking. Many people before me have tried similar things; what I am doing differently is considering the subject from a basis of ethics. Bringing ethics into a subject where it had not been applied before can often make the subject look different; it is this which I will attempt here.

I believe that ethics is essentially about power and how power is used, and that also means the power to believe in oneself and one's own worth. Nursing needs to empower itself if it is to have an identity, and using ethics as a basis may be one way forward; it is not the only way, but it is a part of the way at this moment. I hope that, by sharing a little of my vision, this book will contribute to the wider identity of nursing's future.

I am writing in the style of 'we' and 'us' even though I have not been a practising nurse for many years now. As a teacher, editor and writer, I am, however, still in the field of nursing, and here I am concerned as much with the world-wide concept of nursing as a profession as with individual practitioners. It is in this sense that I still consider myself a nurse and write as one of them.

As this is a book of ideas, it is not specific to any grade or category of nurses nor indeed only to nurses. Students on Project 2000 courses might find it helpful in their studies of professional identity, and nurses who are qualified might get some ideas for expanding their horizons. Students of ethics might find it useful in looking at ethics from a different angle. I hope too that other health professionals might be stimulated in thinking further in their own areas so that barriers can be broken down and partnerships created.

This book is the result of several years' thinking and talking with many people. New ideas have constantly presented themselves, changing and shaping this book. I am particularly indebted to friends, colleagues and students in many different settings. They are too numerous to mention by name, but I hope that any who read this book will know themselves to be acknowledged and thanked. As editor of the journal *Nursing Ethics,* I am in the privileged position of reading all the articles, often several times over, which makes me familiar with much material on ethics. The contact with authors, and especially with my editorial board and consultant colleagues, pushes me also into wider visions of the possible and the practical. I am grateful to them for their insights and support.

A special thank you goes to the person who gave me permission to use the psychiatrist's story in Chapter 1.

My particular gratitude, however, goes to Lady Helen Oppenheimer, whose ideas I have used as a basis for this book and whose comments on an early draft were not only helpful and insightful, but also humorous and highly pertinent.

The conversations (and delicious meals) with the Reverend Dr Michael and Mrs Jean Wilson in their home in Birmingham have been highlights whenever they were possible. The Wilsons have given of their generosity of spirit and their time more than they could possibly imagine, and my deepest thanks go to them. Michael's ideas in particular have been influential in the last chapter.

Last but not least, a sincere thank you is also extended to the two reviewers of the manuscript and to Richenda Milton-Thompson, publisher at Macmillan, for her unfailing support in seeing this project through the many changes and developments.

VERENA TSCHUDIN

1

Nurses Matter

When a politician says that nurses matter, nurses are at first pleased and then recognise it as a gimmick. When a patient says it, nurses know it is true. When nurses say it to themselves, their heads perhaps agree, but their hearts and their gut feelings speak of a different experience. If nurses are to matter, they have to persuade these three constituencies in equal measure.

Nurses matter

The title of this book and this chapter aim to enforce the very basic idea that nurses matter, in particular that their work matters. We do not need to make excuses or feel somewhat ashamed for being 'only' nurses. In the next chapter, I will be considering the ethical ideas behind the statement that 'people matter', but here I want to start with the fundamental notion that nurses matter as people; what we do matters; what we contribute matters; what we say matters; what we believe matters; what we think and feel matters; what we are matters; and it matters that our voice is heard and considered.

Very often, when reading articles or chapters written by nurses on the distinctive contribution made by nurses and nursing, I detect an air of being surprised by what we can achieve. It is not said in so many words, but, compared with the style of such writing by other professionals, a kind of uncertainty is detectable and a lack of self-assurance can be sensed: 'I am just a nurse.' There are many reasons why this feeling comes across, not least being my own projection and understanding. Somehow, I believe, however, that I am not alone in picking up such sentiments.

That nurses matter is the fundamental message of this book; what the message is in detail will be considered in each chapter. I start off here with a more general overview by considering the three main protagonists on this stage.

The politician, the patient and the nurse

In any kind of public service industry, there is an inevitable tension between the users (patients, clients and customers), those who pay for and direct the service (national and local government) and the service givers in this case, nurses. To satisfy all three dimensions is never easy; in particular, service givers find it hard to consider themselves as equally important as service users. As every nurse knows, the three elements are completely interrelated, but I will consider first the forces of control, which are often sources of conflict and mistrust.

The politician

All over the world, people have come to mistrust politicians, managers and policy makers, or any kind of authority for that matter. Too often, their words and their actions have not coincided. Their promises have sounded enticing at the time, but a few months down the line, the reality is different. When nurses have become politicians and leaders, we accuse them of losing touch with the reality (Kenny, 1998, p. 12). We see them playing the power games, and we dismiss them. If we meet them at a conference or gathering, we notice how they congregate with their peers rather than with those who used to be their colleagues. If we do manage to catch their eye, they excuse themselves, having to have a word with someone more important. They are not 'one of us' any longer; we are not 'one of them'.

If gaps are so quickly created, how is it possible to persuade politicians that 'they' and 'we' are not pulling in the opposite direction, do not speak a different language and have different aims? That we are not different people? By politicians, I mean here not only Members of Parliament, but the many movers and shakers of our society and system of health care. I am applying the term 'politicians' very loosely and generally.

The new millennium seems to be a symbol for change and transition in every sphere of life. We are increasingly aware of the interconnectedness of all things, yet, in contrast, also of the increasing personalisation of everything. Such opposing forces will, do and need to clash if they are to be clarified and enriched. However, they are not simply opposite forces that, like two armies of old, are trying to destroy one another. This sort of warfare is no longer applicable, but the forces have not diminished. We cannot apply the old measures and understanding to the new situations; we need to find new ways of interpreting what is happening. This demands imagination, vision and openness (see Chapter 6). It also demands some sort of anchor – some firm basis or ground that is solid and against which we can test something. However, few things in life are immovable and so primary that everyone recognises them as valid. The philosophers have attempted to name them, religions have made them sacred, and lawyers constantly try to define them, yet these are the very forces and authorities that we question.

Nursing is certainly not alone in the struggle for acknowledgement and importance. Groups of people, professions and whole sections of society are fighting for their livelihood, but nursing's background makes it peculiarly vulnerable in this race for a place in the sun. It is not only that nurses have been women, and therefore subordinate for generations. The work of nurses – care and caring – has to do with bodies, especially diseased bodies. In a world where the young and the beautiful are idolised, the old, the worn and the unhealthy, who are generally those who need care, do not have much attraction. Nurses deal day in and day out with bodies, particularly with what comes out of them, which generally smells and is unsightly, so that they become linked with sights, smells and sounds that people tend to avoid. Our Western culture has demeaned the body (by idolising it) and therefore those who look after bodies; hence, the pay of those who work with bodies is low (Lawler, 1991, pp. 44–52). The care receivers are frequently also either infants or tend to be infantilised (Tronto, 1993, p. 170), diminishing the role of the care givers even further.

In today's world, the task of nurses and nursing is no longer to say, especially to medical colleagues, 'Excuse me, sir, can I help you?', but to say, 'All our tasks centre on this person here, who is made vulnerable through illness. Both our contributions are needed. Neither is more important than the other, or better or worse than the other: they are simply different. *Vive la différence*, and the difference I make is vital.'

In this setting, it often seems impossible to meet politicians, managers and policy makers on an equal footing. They are not inclined to listen to talk of caring for diseased bodies and how nurses perceive their own and their patients' feelings and emotions, as well as the 'significant impact on nursing practice' (Mazhindu, 1998, p. 28) they have. Those who run the health services have to be concerned with facts and figures, with managing the institution and with getting results.

The different languages that politicians and nurses speak means that they are likely never to hear what the other is saying or, if they hear the words, they do not understand what is being referred to. Many people (for example Gilligan, 1982; Noddings, 1984; Tschudin, 1992; Tronto, 1993) have argued that an ethic of care is the best criterion for making health care more accessible and human. This, however, would demand that politicians change their stance, and this is unlikely. Tronto (1993, p. 172) advises 'a recommitment to democratic processes, for example *listening* [emphasis added] and to including care-receivers in determining the process of care'. She goes on to say that 'caring is best understood not as a utopian device that will end all conflict, but as a value that should be made more central in our constellation of political concerns'.

It is clear that 'caring' has moved more centrally with the emphasis on holistic care, but it is also clear that anyone who is not daily surrounded by the sheer practicalities of caring cannot comprehend their overwhelming presence, need and drain on human resources. Politicians need their distance in order to manage and organise. They cannot get involved with details of suffering, which is always personal, private and totally unique.

However, it also seems that many accounts of nurses showing how effective they are, simply in terms of money, are not taken enough into consideration by the powers that be. Watson (1993) details some figures:

In 12 out of 14 areas the nurse practitioner care was rated higher than physician care, including services that depend on communication with patients and preventive action. (US Congress Office of Technological Assessment, 1986)

The US would save $6.4 billion to $8.75 billion in health care costs each year, if the barriers [that] nurse practitioners face were removed. (*Wall Street Journal*, 1993)

Better utilisation of nursing and nurses in Canada is tied to what could be the '12 billion dollar solution' to health costs. (Rachlis and Kushner, 1989)

Despite '30 years of cost-effective data on nurses as primary care providers; despite dramatic 40 percent drops in premature birth rates when nurse-midwives provide prenatal care to disadvantaged populations' (Huey, 1988), controls against nursing practice have persisted. (Watson, 1993, p. 5)

Similar examples, too numerous to mention, abound in the UK and other parts of the world, of nurses either now having or potentially having significant impacts on health and on budgets (if they were given the chance). But they are not given the chance, and the thorny question of why remains.

I do not want to repeat the many arguments surrounding this topic; they are too well known. My contention is that, despite impressive figures, nurses have never yet managed to persuade the politicians of their case. Politicians know what they want and need but seem to imply that nursing cannot give it to them. Nursing *has* got what politicians want and need, but nurses have not yet convinced politicians of this, *because nurses have not yet been convinced of it themselves*. I believe that nursing needs to have confidence in its own validity and that this is a crucial element. Nurses do care, but an ethic of care is not enough to give nurses and nursing the credibility that makes care legitimate. Such an ethic is more divisive and exclusive than strengthening and inclusive. A more inclusive ethic based on more general principles may be more effective in bridging the gap between 'them' and 'us', between politicians and nurses. I will attempt to describe this in this book.

The Patient

Many of the ethical problems in care are created because various professional groups vie with each other for superiority – for who has the moral high ground. This is largely a problem of labour division in health care, but it becomes expressed in moral and ethical terms (Chambliss, 1996, p. 181). The recipients of care, and the pawns in this power game, are always the patients and clients. They are the losers. When power and drive come to a point of conflict, the weakest part is affected. This is why patients have to depend on nurses so much. For nurses:

> there can be no quick review of lab reports, a scribbling of orders, and then a fast exit down the hall. Nurses carry out the scribbled orders, deliver the medications, pass the food trays, monitor the IVs and the ventilators. Nurses give baths, catheterize patients, turn patients who cannot move themselves, clean bedsores, change soiled sheets, and constantly watch patients, writing notes on their patients' progress or deterioration. (Chambliss, 1996, p. 64)

Patients have every reason to say that nurses matter. Good, bad or indifferent care affects their health and their whole existence. Patients remember nurses for years, whereas they may not remember other health professionals.

Because of the way in which health care is organised, someone – usually someone who is paid – has to do the practical caring. Those who are ill need help, and our high-tech ways of making people better mean that they need a great deal of technically competent help. People who are dependent on machines for their life are doubly dependent: on the machine and on the nurses who watch and control the machines. The very helplessness of patients in situations of extreme vulnerability means that nurses play a vital role. The fact that this is not simply 'doing to' but 'being with' (Campbell, 1984, p. 48) also makes nurses vulnerable. They use their own selves therapeutically via the relationship that is created through caring. To the person who is dependent on the nurse, it matters how an injection is given: not simply competently but with that touch which implies that the injection is going to help. Much of nursing can be considered as a delivery of tasks, but patients can tell when a task is given with care or is 'just' routine. When patients are considered in this way, they respond and co-operate, thus maintaining the relationship.

> Nurses not only care, but also share. They share themselves, their skills, their knowledge. They share the journey with the client, perhaps intimately. They are there when people are born and when they die – surely the two most intimate events in the life of a human being.

Being present at one's daughter's birthing is nevertheless very different from being present at a client's birthing; being present when a loved one dies is different from being present at a patient's death. Our patients and clients are like our mothers or sons, and when we care for relative strangers, we care for a person who matters to us. All nurses do their caring and sharing personally; this is part of the satisfaction and also the cost of nursing. Neither should be underestimated.

Patients and clients are the nurses' best allies. From the point of view of health care generally, and the kind of health care needed in the future, it is absolutely necessary that patients no longer have images of angels and play-objects, ladies with lamps or sergeant major-type matrons. For this to happen, nurses themselves have to change their image. Nurses who hide their feelings and take on personas while they work do not help patients to understand that more than just 'ministering' is going on. Nurses not only care, but also share, and this is an extremely important part of their work. They share their knowledge, themselves and their feelings. Only by using themselves therapeutically can they claim to be professionals. By this, I do not mean wearing their hearts on their sleeves but sharing their humanity with their clients so that clients will know that they count and have been heard, understood and valued. Nurses will then know that they have made a significant contribution to the welfare of a person, and, in so doing, they have contributed to their own health and welfare, satisfaction and personal and emotional growth. Humanity depends on sharing. Patients know this when they are ill, and in order to use the experience of illness as positively as possible, nurses have to understand this important fact and use it, making it known that they do, and also being proud of it.

Patients do not have to be persuaded that nurses matter: they depend on them. This means that nurses also have to take their role as advocates more seriously. It is not only the individual person who has to have his or her rights respected: patients also need to understand that nurses often have to fight for the environment to be as healthy as possible for all concerned, especially patients. In several countries, nurses have gone on strike for better pay and conditions. While striking is a very delicate subject (see Chapter 7), patients and clients are often very ready to support nurses in their actions: they know that they will indirectly be the beneficiaries. Bickley (1997, p. 308) states that, in New Zealand, 'the public sees nurses as defenders of the health services', and Katsuragi (1997, p. 316) tells of nurses at Keio University Hospital in Tokyo who 'collected over 2000 signatures every day from the patients' in support of the 'Nurse Wave' movement, which campaigned for better working conditions for nurses and better health care.

It is possible that patients support nurses out of pity – nurses have a terrible job – or out of self-interest as they depend on nurses. Motives are never simple and obvious. If we want patients to assert that nurses matter, we have to ensure that patients know what the real work of nursing is, that they appreciate it and that they do so with more than a box of chocolates. This means that we have to educate patients by sharing with them ourselves and our work, forming a partnership that will find the 'them' and 'us' division arbitrary. However, nurses have to believe in the first place that they need, can and do share and that this is the ethical way forward. This will be further considered in Chapter 9.

The Nurse

Ethics and morality are the driving forces of all care, and ethics is as much about 'what is' as about 'what can (or may) be'. To be ethical persons, we have to be concerned about the future and how to improve practice. Nurses have a drive to make people better and therefore to leave humanity generally in a better (or healthier) position than they found it in. Their very practice is future orientated. The energy that they invest in this care is, however, rarely used with the same vigour for improving the lot of nurses themselves; on the contrary, much of their energy goes into moaning, which can create an atmosphere of helplessness bordering on despair. However, good care in an unhealthy or bad environment is only half good, and nursing is about the environment of care as much as about care itself. If we feel uncomfortable or unhealthy in our working environment, or if our conditions are far from ideal, our work itself is a contradiction. We cannot give to others what we have not got: if we are not cared for we cannot care; if we are not supported, we cannot support others; if our relationships with colleagues are dismal, our relationships with clients will not be much better (see Chapter 8).

Nurses matter – immensely, intensely and supremely. It is not just that doctors and nurses could not do their work without each other. Patients could not be without nurses, at least as the labour divisions are at the moment. I am convinced that such divisions will change enormously over the next 20 or 30 years (see Chapter 6). What the role of nurses and nursing will be depends on what nurses themselves are willing and able to imagine and apply. Nurses matter at the most basic level of such changes. Nurses matter because their experience of caring has accumulated and is now a fund on which to draw. This fund is like a magic mountain: it does not diminish, but each time we make use of it, it grows bigger still because experience is cumulative.

This mountain of experience is not only nursing's great asset, but also its stumbling block. It has helped nursing to make itself felt as a profession by providing much of the research that was necessary to make nursing credible. In so doing, nursing, at least in the UK, has been able to hide behind this mountain, believing that other professions will see that the mountain is there and take it seriously. If nurses today are not heard or taken seriously, part of the problem is that for too long they have dismissed the importance of this mountain of experience, and when they now ask others to take them seriously, they seem to wonder why it is not happening.

Chambliss (1996, p. 75) says that 'if there is a single dominant theme in nurses' complaints about their work, it is the lack of respect they feel, from lay persons, from co-workers, and especially from physicians'. Nurses have not yet reached the summit of their own mountain. It remains a mountain of experience only and is not yet a mountain from which to survey the landscape, one on which to stand and feel secure: a mountain that many people will want to climb, which is one in a range of mountains, all equally important and beautiful, and which is the headquarters of action for change. Nurses have not yet learned that by inviting people, in particular politicians, to come and visit their mountain, it will not disappear, but that people will instead learn to appreciate the view and wonder why they had never made the trek before. Mountains are also places where people have visions, not just of the landscape, but also of inner insights. Nursing and nurses need to recognise that their mountain of (practical) experience is also a mountain of visionary experience. They need to become much more thoroughly and daringly familiar with the possibilities of their mountain and the various images and symbols offered there. Nurses generally have not trusted their own sense of importance enough.

It is this sense of security, confidence and importance that nursing has to (re)gain. This has to happen for nursing as a profession, but it can only be achieved by the work of individual nurses. *Nurses* matter, and they can make *nursing* matter.

At every point, nursing and nurses seem to be a long way away from an equality in leadership that shapes the future of health care. Some people wonder if there could ever be equality or indeed if this is a good and reasonable goal. Maybe we do not need equality with medicine or physiotherapy and the many other professions on which people rely when they are ill. When each profession feels secure in itself, there is no need for competition, and each can make its own contribution, respecting that of others and not glancing over its shoulder to see what others are doing or having to defend itself morally and practically. Each of the professions in health care has something different to offer. Like mountains in a range, they belong to each other but cannot take the other's place. Nursing has to learn that its mountain is as important as its neighbour but that it perhaps needs a little help from its 'tourist board' to advertise its strength, beauty and significance: it needs to be put on the map by nurses themselves.

Confidence in the self

Another metaphor from nature is that of rivers: rivers can only flow because their source is on a solid (and unmoveable) mountain. All great rivers start with little springs. Everything of value starts with a single thought, a single coin, a single gesture. It is through the accumulation of the thoughts, coins and gestures that great works have been accomplished. In the same way, it is possible to say that individuals have changed the world by the way in which they have acted, allowing others to act in the same way. One can mention any great religious and spiritual leader: Moses, Buddha, Jesus, Mohammed. Nearer to our time, Mahatma Gandhi, Martin Luther King and Mother Teresa have started movements that have enabled millions of people to find meaning and expression. We cannot all be world leaders so it is good also to acknowledge those among us who have made a difference in our personal lives, in whatever way. They may be teachers, community leaders or business people. Their effectiveness in changing the world may be less dramatic, but to acknowledge them matters. Every one of us knows of a nurse who has made or is making an imortant impact on our lives; we should be more generous with our praise and thanks to our friends.

Too often we hear horror stories about hospitals and about treatment and care that have gone wrong. Those who have stories of success, kindness and excellence to tell stand out. Is it really that only bad news *is* news? We cannot affirm each other with negative news, and unlike the case with steel, beating people does not make them better. If we want to help people to get better, we have to feel good about ourselves first, otherwise we do not have the right conditions in which to practise holistic care.

Nothing builds success like success. We need what Handy (1997) calls 'proper selfishness' (see Chapter 7). He explains that this means a proper concern with ourselves that searches for the reality that we are. This inevitably means being intertwined with people. Our own self-respect, Handy (1997, p. 87) says, really only comes from a responsibility for people and things. Success makes us properly selfish, and being successful only happens in relation to people and things.

If we matter as nurses, we experience this as people, but this takes form only in relation to our clients and colleagues. There was a time when we thought that telling nurses they *would* never make a nurse would make them one, that not getting involved with patients would shelter nurses from trauma, and that by sparing nurses from decision making they could get on with their jobs better. In every situation, the contrary has been proved. It is only by getting involved that we can use our professional judgement, by being part of the planning that we can take pride in our work and by getting our backs stroked that we can feel worthwhile.

All the self-assertion training in the world will not help if we cannot put it into practice. If we, as nurses, are to make an impact on the world around us and in the wider professional sphere, we have to start with ourselves. We *are* OK – and so are our colleagues. This does not mean perfectionism. Everyone makes mistakes, and there is much that we can learn from our mistakes. The waltz, that gracious dance, works on the principle of two steps forwards or sideways and one step back. The steps back are important in the movement. A proper selfishness can acknowledge setbacks and mistakes, learn from them and even see them as part of the overall picture. The steps forward build on the steps backwards or sideways. They are also the steps necessary for self-reflection. The important thing is that there is movement, and that in itself is assertive. We need to build on this and believe in ourselves.

Reflective practice has been widely used in nursing in recent times to learn the art and science of the profession (Andrews *et al.*, 1998, pp. 413–17). A similar process needs to be applied to the profession itself and also by individual nurses in order to feel deep within themselves the confidence to be equals with their professional colleagues. Not only in New Zealand, but also world-wide, must the public see nurses as the defenders of the health services. We cannot leave it to others to acknowledge this role, but we must do it ourselves. The vital need is for confidence in our own ability and the truth and justice of our message. The energy that easily goes into bewailing the state of affairs has to be channelled into a positive move to improve it.

Nurses matter, we matter, you matter, I matter. The fact that we actually have to tell ourselves this fundamental reality reveals how much we doubt it as a profession. When I am with nurses, I know that we believe in this fundamental truth, but when I am with a mixed group of health professionals, I sense that this truth seems to buckle at the knees and we no longer fundamentally believe it. When we acknowledge both the truth that we matter and the fact that we doubt it when other health professionals are present, we can take the appropriate steps to change this message that we tend to convey – that others are OK but we are not.

Many nurses are galvanised into action only after some event that has left them angry at the treatment they have received or at being disregarded, sidelined or simply dismissed as unimportant. Perhaps most people need some trigger before they take action on their own behalf. We generally only know the values by which we live when they are questioned by an unexpected personal or global event. A TV picture spurs us into action, a demeaning treatment makes us realise that we have been dehumanised. We need to do something to restore the damage. This in itself gives us the energy necessary.

It need not only be world-shattering events that give us the drive and clear-sightedness for action. It is often a very small incident that touches a raw nerve. When we are aware of the possibility *for* action, we are more acutely attuned to the possibilities *of* action. Acting when confronted with a challenge then becomes the ethical stance or imperative. Acting ethically is one of the things by which we will be judged. Even more basic than ethical action, feeding the confidence in ourself is a moral action, touching the self at the roots. It is from that depth that we have to believe in our actions as nurses because the future of humanity depends on it.

The ethic of care

The ethic of care has been essential to nursing since the early 1980s, but it it has never been fully accepted as a theory in its own right (Gallagher, 1995; Rickard *et al.*, 1996). It has been in opposition to an ethic of justice, and comparisons have been made, trying to justify the one or the other. More recently, authors have acknowledged that it should not represent an either/or stance but a both/and one because the theories stress different aspects and thus complement each other (Churchill, 1994; Norberg and Udén, 1995; Kuhse, 1997). I believe that the acknowledgement of an ethic of care has helped nursing to take a leap forward that would have been impossible without it. I am concerned here with the step before the theory: the people, events and motives that give the theory validity.

An ethic of care is characterised by 'receptivity, relatedness and responsiveness' and 'begins with the moral attitude or longing for goodness and not with moral reasoning' (Noddings, 1984, p. 2). I believe that it is this longing for goodness that is the basic motivation for most people who go into nursing. However, in their education and in working in institutional settings, nurses learn to accept the values of reasoning as desirable above all else, and thus a moral conflict is created. Believing – personally and professionally – that goodness, compassion, personal engagement and covenant relationships are equally as valid as logic gets relegated. Nurses begin to believe that their motives were 'wrong' to begin with, and this leads to a loss of confidence in their moral stance and hence in their ability to stand by their basic convictions. We need to recover this basic conviction and value; only then can we make use of it. Nurses instinctively know of thousands of ways in which to seek and bring 'goodness' to individual people, and of many, many world-wide needs for appropriate care.

Noddings (1984, p. 2) points out that, when faced with a dilemma, 'women ask for more information'. It is the need for telling our stories that is basic. Whether it be a happy event or a sad one, we need to express ourselves and tell our stories in order to make sense of the events in our lives. We need to tell our story again and again, and in this way to reach the core or meaning of what is happening. We need to share our experiences for them to become meaningful. It is only in the context of relationships and community that we become humanised.

Telling stories is essential in reflective practice. What is important, however, is that we listen to the essence of what the person is saying rather than to what we want to hear. The patient who says, 'I am scared of this operation' is not heard if she gets an answer like, 'You'll be alright; this sort of operation is routine here and you have a good surgeon.' The patient needs to tell her story of fear: what the fear is, when it started, why it started and where it has led her. In stories of human suffering, we need to hear not so much the practical details as the untold and perhaps not yet understood meaning. In doing this, we are carrying out the essential work of any ethic: being receptive, relating to the other and responding in the most fitting way. In listening to others, we are sharing and expressing that we are 'with' them. In sharing, we become equal, and this allows us to be moral.

As we do this to others, we need to do it to ourselves. Nursing has long been telling its story; telling the history of nursing has now become trendy. An analysis of the gender issues in nursing has filled many pages of articles and dissertations, but the deep cry of nursing for an understanding of its need to express itself in an ethical manner has, I contend, hardly been heard yet. Not that it has not been tried, but nursing itself and nurses themselves have to respond to their own need first. When nurses believe that their cry for relevance and for being heard is real and valid, they can then address more clearly the demands of people everywhere, and their work then becomes ethical. That this cry is heard, responded to and taken seriously is a matter of justice. It is a basic element of human justice that we hear each other's stories.

When we assert that nurses care, we are also prone to asserting that we 'do' something to others rather than that we 'are' something with others. I believe that one of the reasons why an ethic of care has never been completely accepted is because it has this tendency to separate and exclude. This can make the proponents of the theory defensive and lead to deeper divisions. In saying that nursing works with an ethic of care, there is additionally a hint of a sense of duty: an ethic of care is imposed on nurses, it is something that we ought to do or assent to. There are many duties in life that are not only reasonable, but also beneficial and taken on willingly. Perhaps, as with much of knowledge, an ethic of care in nursing has run its course, and new insights and views are making themselves felt. The principle that 'people matter' is a more normative statement, without the sense of 'ought' about it. It

is more an 'of course' statement because it comes from a
different angle. It feels less heavy and imposed, and more simply
a fact that cannot be ignored. It is inclusive. It gives us the
sense that we are equal to other health care professionals. We
do not have to assert ourselves before we can be taken seriously. When we know that we matter, we give out different vibes:
those of a fundamental 'OK-ness'. An ethic that is inclusive
and egalitarian is more acceptable. It tends to lessen the divisions between care givers and care receivers. It is this which
I will address in the following three chapters.

In my own defence, I need to make it clear that I do not
want to contradict those who are far more knowledgeable than
I am on matters of theories and concepts. The tenor of this
book is one of search and vision rather than dogmatism. I have
benefited from an ethic of care in my thinking and teaching,
and need to acknowledge this debt. In the context of this book,
I am proposing that another approach and idea might now
take nursing and nurses another stretch of the journey.

Making a difference

A look at any professional journal will demonstrate how nurses
make a difference in the lives of sick and ill people. Increasingly, nurses also have to think of and be in the forefront of
preventive care, not only in the developing world, but in the
developed world too. Our resources have to be more adequately
managed and more justly distributed.

'Nurses could be the key to positive patient outcomes',
according to Vaughan (1996), who refers to 'a study showing
better patient outcomes in nurse-led versus medical-led units'.
She says that the outcomes surprised many and that money is
now being sought to discover what nurses did to generate such
positive results. The answer, she feels, is the 'caring relationship between nurse and patient'. These are not isolated studies
and findings, and only complement those quoted above. What
Vaughan has drawn attention to are the relationships that
matter. It is not good management, enough resources or a stable
environment, but that most intangible and unmeasurable
element – the human contact – that seems to be the lynch-pin.

An ethic in which 'people matter' is fundamental is very heavily based on the reality of relationships.

What such remarks and studies show is how vitally important care and human contact are. To be effective, care has to be delivered by a human person; that is, qualified nurses matter. Vaughan's study, however, is certainly not the first to come to this conclusion, but this acknowledgement still does not seem to make much of a difference. I believe that it will only make a difference when nurses themselves begin to put this into such ethical and political language so that it cannot but be heard and taken seriously. Nurses need to say their piece in such a way that it can be understood by politicians, patients and themselves in no other way. Some of the language in the next three chapters may point in a direction that can be helpful to nurses in their drive to be heard by others and, above all, to hear themselves.

2

People Matter

That people matter is the basis of all ethical behaviour. Because caring for people is the *raison d'être* of nurses and nursing, the basic belief of nurses and nursing is that people matter. How and why people matter has been the concern of philosophers down the ages, but it is increasingly also the concern of all those who work in health care, especially nurses. Issues of human rights, scarce resources and how to reconcile the two have to be addressed far more deeply and intimately than ever before. The contribution of nurses and nursing to this debate is crucial because any answers given will affect us all. It is therefore important that nurses have an ethical basis from which to argue. This chapter intends to help in clarifying why 'people matter'.

The phrase 'nurses matter' is at once the vision and the message, the present and the future. All the various implicit and explicit aspects of such a slogan need to be considered, and this can mean walking around the subject before arriving at an overall view. This chapter consists of such a 'walk' in the general direction of philosophical starting points.

The basic message that nursing gives out is that people matter. Because people matter, they need the best care possible when sick or ill, or vulnerable for any reason. Nurses can and do give that care – there is no question about that – but too often their care is hampered by misunderstandings and misconceptions, as well as by policies over which nurses have no control. This diminishes not only nurses as professionals, but also the dignity of patients and clients. When people no longer matter – or do not matter as much as they should – it becomes a professional imperative to redress the trend towards inhumanity. If nurses want to broadcast the message, they have to base this on an ethic arguing that people matter.

Harris (1973) says that the final position in transactional analysis is 'I'm OK – You're OK' and that this is reached by a conscious and verbal decision. Only when we can understand that we are truly OK can we also accept that others are OK. Harris says that 'we do not drift into [this] new position. It is a decision we make. In this respect it is like a conversion experience' (Harris, 1973, p. 49). By considering the ways in which people matter, I hope to outline some of the elements that could help us to reach this point of 'conversion'.

In this and the following two chapters, I am using the ideas of Helen Oppenheimer (1995), who has an engaging way of using concepts and language to make age-old concepts accessible in her thesis of 'mattering'. Oppenheimer herself did not want to define what 'mattering' is – not in order to be contrary, but because she believes that it is a basic concept such as 'good' or 'person' and is best not defined. Her starting point is simply that each of us can truly say 'I matter'.

People matter

Today I committed myself to life. I committed myself to no suicide and to no hospital. I am proud of myself that I've got through another day and I'm still alive tonight and ready to say something. Long days go by when I'm completely and utterly mute. I can't string three words together. It is exciting again to have something to say, not just something to think. I am writing to you, people like me, who get trapped in a prison of unsolicited silence. I am so jealous of all those around me who seem simply to be getting on with their lives; buying tomatoes, getting on buses and making phone calls. These simple everyday movements seem to herald an ability which escapes me at present; to be intentioned, determined, able to cope and to make decisions. I have been drifting for months, wanting to curl up in bed and disappear. I think of the thousands of people who, like me, feel like a living corpse. This phenomenon is almost impossible to communicate. It is unlike any I have ever known personally. Professionally I have seen it but not until now understood it from its underbelly. This lack of understanding brings some shame to me as I am a psychotherapist and have been for twenty years. Until now I have not known the true meaning of clinical depression.

What broke the silence? I laughed with old friends tonight for the first time in months. I saw a psychiatrist... who, with love in his

eyes, said 'I'd like to see you again'. What penetrated my thick
armour was the caring in his eyes when he spoke to me, saying 'I
know you are in a depression but I take all that into the invitation
to want to see you again'. What enormous kindness. R.D. Laing
once said 'Treatment is the way you treat people'. I felt well treated
even though I was not the specimen of humanity every mother
wishes for. (personal communication)

This story epitomises many of the aspects that health care
workers meet every day:

- the helplessness of the patient
- the 'knowing and not knowing': even as professionals
  ourselves, we cannot know what suffering is like until we
  experience it ourselves
- the need to tell our story
- the need to be acknowledged personally and as a unique
  human being
- the need to be loved
- the need to be supported
- the need not to be judged.

Our patients and clients meet and need these things, and
we as carers meet and need them. When they are not there,
we suffer, and illness of one kind or another ensues. This is
the story of patients, but it is also particularly the story of
nurses and nursing. Looking at some of its aspects may be
painful, but every nurse knows that, in order to get better, we
often have to go through pain.

When using the term 'people matter' in a nursing context,
the assumption is easily made that this applies to patients and
clients, and indeed it does. However, it applies equally to nurses
and any professionals who care for patients and clients. 'People
matter' is therefore an inclusive term, and any examples used
may apply sometimes to patients and clients, and sometimes
to nurses.

It is at times of crisis that our values are sharpened. Most
people will have experienced some time of crisis when they
became aware of who their true friends are. They are the ones
who supported them, stood by them and did not judge them,
with whom they could cry and in whose company they could

be angry or out of control. Suffering is often talked about or reported on a massive scale, but for each person, there is the individual experience. There may be hundreds of people sick in a hospital, but we can only be aware of the personal suffering of a few of them. It is the person who matters, but the people are our concern. The tension between the one and the many, the individual and society, will always exercise our ethical minds, as well as our personal and moral behaviour. Not to acknowledge that tension can lead to the devastating situations so well known in nursing where different groups pursue different ideals. Because a person matters, people matter.

That *people* matter seems to be a given fact. Many people would argue today that people, animals, trees, the earth generally and the environment in particular all matter equally because all depend on each other. It can also be said that, if we care for one of these, by implication we also care for the others. As so much of nursing is about preventive care, nurses also need to be concerned with global issues as they clearly affect health in the much wider sense than simply the small sphere of our personal influence. The interaction between the very personal and the global has to be increasingly our concern, and nursing has to become much more aware of the impact of the drop of water in the ocean and of the natural cycle that this creates.

Perhaps most of us have speculated what it might be like to be Queen or Prime Minister, or some other famous person. Would we do what the real holder of that office or fame does? What would we do differently, and why? How would we influence the world? What would we do to make it better? What do we mean by 'better'? Such speculation can reveal our hidden drives and urges, in particular our values. Equally, identifying who our hero is and saying or noting why will tell us not only what we admire in an other person but what we already are or have in the way of personal attributes but perhaps dare not use or acknowledge. To stay with that thought for a moment may give us more instant self-awareness and self-assurance than perhaps a lengthy course of discussion might. It may reveal our personal basis for the assertion that people matter. The personal shapes the global, and the global becomes the personal again.

All our lives are concerned with people. Every one of us has to consider what matters to us, and that cannot be done in isolation. Whatever we do impacts on other people sooner or later. How we treat ourselves in private is an indication of how we are likely to treat others, and how we treat others mirrors how we treat ourselves.

The NHS sometimes gives the impression that it would run very smoothly were it not for the patients. They make impossible demands, and their unforeseen behaviour throws budgets off line. When we forget that the NHS, or any other health care system, functions only because of people, nurses in particular need to remind themselves of their advocacy role. The primacy of patients and clients has to be an absolute. More clearly still, it is the individual person who counts, not someone with the label 'patient', for that is ultimately what 'people matter' means.

When we assert that 'people matter', we assert also that the whole person matters. We cannot then say that people matter as long as they are under 70, don't abuse the system, don't make impossible demands (patients), don't demand too much, don't get hurt or injured and remain 'reasonable' with their requests (nurses). 'People matter' is a positive statement, and to carry it through, we cannot then put negative stops against it, otherwise we create injustice at every turn. Indeed, 'people matter' is a strong protagonist for justice. This is not the justice that says that Peter and Paul have to have exactly the same – Peter and Paul are not the same person with the same needs, but both deserve to be equally respected and listened to. Only in this way can we determine the needs (rather than the wants) of each and respond to them.

'Curved cucumbers'

The concept that people matter has to be made applicable and practical. People matter, but people are also selfish and not the specimen of humanity every mother wishes for. This inherent state of selfishness has been described by St Augustine (AD 354–430) as 'being curved in upon oneself'. Always quick to apply metaphors to everyday objects, Oppenheimer (1995, p. 63) likens this state to that of her own home-grown cucumbers, which are curved rather than straight. Writing from a Christian standpoint, she goes on to say that 'Christianity is about how we can be unbent'. This is probably true of every religious system, as well as of therapies and psychological interventions of many kinds. Just as babies are born with their fingers turned inwards into a fist, life loosens this curving inwards until, at death, our hands are open and limp. In that process, we are not only becoming more 'properly selfish' and truly human ourselves, but, as we do, are also enabling those around us to be more 'properly selfish' and human too; similarly, we are affected by their efforts at humanising their environment.

The polarisation into people who seem supremely confident in their abilities and those who lack any such confidence is becoming more obvious. People who are confident in their abilities tend to come across as selfish and those who lack confidence as undecided and wet – at least in specific instances and relationships. Both can be described as lacking in psychological maturity. Much of this arises from nature, but much also derives from nurture; in other words, much of it is beyond our control. However, when we apply 'people matter' to situations that are seemingly uncontrollable, we give a positive message, and what seemed impossible can become possible. Being out of control is not all there is to it. We do not simply have to stay with our curves and misfortunes. We can indeed become 'OK'. Once we realise this, not only do we *become* OK, but also we *are* OK. The basic belief in ourselves – the 'proper selfishness' – enables us to believe in our vision, message and means of communicating them.

It may be argued that health care exists in order to straighten what has become bent, but the problem is that health care is concerned with bodies whereas the metaphor applies to the psyche and the personality. When considering the idea of 'respect for the person' as an ethical principle, the issue becomes more difficult, and we are into the area of professional control, persuasion and legislation. How much can we persuade a person that his or her views are 'wrong'? When is someone capable of giving consent to treatment, and what may be the circumstances that might change this? How is 'superior' professional knowledge used?

These questions point to the problem that constantly arises in health care when considering only a part of a person: we treat the diseased organ rather than the person. While this is frowned upon generally, in practice we find it very difficult to think in terms of an individual with unique experiences and needs. When this individual thinks and acts differently from ourselves, or even questions our values, we find it even more difficult to be tolerant and accepting. To what extent is such a person 'curved' and in need of being straightened out? Most of the time this is not a moral question, but when it becomes one, it can quickly lead to major problems. We know of too many situations when a patient did not want to accept some treatment offered and was made to feel guilty with remarks such as 'Do you know what you are doing to your family?' We find it very hard to accept other people's values when this implies not only that they differ from ours, but also that ours are rejected after having been offered in good faith.

> We may need occasionally to ask ourselves whose values are more relevant in given situations. As professionals, our values have been so conditioned by the institution and culture in which we work that to see that *our* values as the more questionable ones may come as a real surprise to many of us.

Wanting (and needing) to fix everything, even when it is not broken, hides a perfectionism that is unhealthy. Gardens without weeds are not gardens but showpieces, cucumbers without curves are artificially grown, and people without peculiar ideas or unexpected beliefs and requests are not 'fully functioning' in that they do not know their own potentiality or are not allowed to exercise it by others. We need our curved cucumbers at all levels while aware that our potential, if by that we mean the human potential, is to be as 'straight' as possible.

What nurses do and say matters immensely, and nurses are often less inclined to impose values or treatments than are their medical colleagues. Because they have more direct contact with patients and clients, they will have heard their stories, and therefore the context for certain ideas or values is more transparent.

This provides a strong argument that nurses need to be much more closely involved in discussions and decision making, as well as in the process of information giving and obtaining consent. Only in this way can we assert that people matter: all people, not just those who fit a certain image or idea.

Assumptions

One of the benefits of a rational mind is that we can quickly make connections with ideas, memories and facts. Such connections prevent us from walking into oncoming cars or prompt us to help someone across the road.

We also make thousands of other helpful and unhelpful connections. A dark blue uniform on a person in the street means 'police', and seeing a patient curled up in a hospital bed with tears running down the cheeks means that something has happened to that person which may need a gentle approach on the part of the nurse. Too often, however, we jump to conclusions that may be many steps further along a line, although these may or may not in fact be there.

When people matter, we need to be careful of the assumptions we make. Seeing a person in a dark blue uniform in the street may lead to the following conclusion: police – I am driving too fast – they will have noticed me – I will be apprehended – I will be fined – I cannot afford it – my driving licence will be endorsed – I am in trouble. Or seeing a patient in bed crying may mean: she has just been given bad news – ('bad' meaning cancer) – she thinks she is dying – she needs to be reassured – I need to do this because I have noticed her – I am no good at this sort of thing – I am a failure (yet again). Or perhaps instead: her husband has just been there – he will have upset her – I do not like that man – he should not talk to her like that – he is an awful person.

Such reasoning goes on all the time, and it is frequently life saving and we are absolutely right. Too often, however, we are not right. We make assumptions about people and events that may at best be harmlessly corrected and at worst may be serious breaches of human rights.

To say that 'people matter' is to say that we respect each other to the extent that we let each other live and do not diminish each other, not even in thought. The kind of argument that I have outlined is typical of our thinking, with its emphasis on guilt, wrongdoing and need for someone to blame. Too often we jump to the negative conclusion, unaware that there might be a positive one, not only about ourselves, but also about other people. It makes us suspicious and lacking in trust in ourselves and others. This inevitably leads to aggressive assertion and deviousness, as well as verbal and physical violence. The negative condition becomes reality simply because we have wished it so: 'I knew I would not get anywhere.'

It is too naïve to imagine that all we have to do is take a positive view of life and all will be well. We cannot change our spots overnight. Communists did not turn into democrats from one day to the next when the Berlin wall came down. If people have not so far mattered in an institution or culture, they cannot matter overnight just because someone says or wishes it to be so. At the basis of any assumption is, however, a simple straight line to a conclusion that may or may not be right. This is rather incredible given that most natural things in life and in nature are not straight but follow more circular or spiral paths. Not even the proverbial bee-line is straight. Would it therefore not be more human and more natural to respond in a similar way, by inviting the other person to tell her or his story, which will, for sure, have many bends and curves in it? What is straight is the view of our eyes: we cannot see round corners. But our lives, like the cucumbers, are curved. Learning to see curved shapes and unusual or different views may therefore be a vital task of living and making sure that people matter.

Making assumptions is clearly helpful in life generally, but making assumptions about people is depriving them of dignity, rights and attention. As nurses, we have taken the role of advocate very seriously in recent times, considering it to be enhancing our professionalism. The difficulty with advocacy is that we can too easily make assumptions: that you know that someone else has not listened; that you know that the client needs help; that you know more and need to help; that you are the right person to help. All these may be facts, but they take much for granted.

When we make assumptions about others, we need to be careful because we can very quickly create barriers between 'them' and 'us', and take away a person's legitimate right to be listened to and understood. We can assume that machines work correctly when we buy them and that our house will be there to come home to, but when we make assumptions about people, we are on shifting ground. We can only base an ethic on the notion that people matter when we put this into practice by listening and hearing what the people say for themselves.

In just the same way, there are many assumptions made about nurses that we all know to be false and degrading. However, we can only challenge these when we make every effort ourselves to let people know that these assumptions are false. We cannot assume that, simply by carrying out our everyday tasks, the population will change its ideas about nurses and nursing. We must believe in the first instance that because we matter as nurses, our story is worth listening to. We cannot assume that because the story is there, people will hear it. Even less can we assume that 'they', having heard the story, will take it seriously and act on it. If we want our vision and message to be relevant, we have to tell it ourselves and put it into action ourselves. In this way, we assert that nurses matter because people matter.

Metamorphosis

In the process of uncurving and growing as human beings, we go through many stages. As so often, these can be described in either/or ways: we lose or gain certainties, beliefs and values. Some people see the negative: isn't it a pity to lose old truths, habits and belief systems? Other people see in it a freedom gained: it can be so liberating to be free of shackling and rigid views, attitudes and outgrown values. At last they are free to express themselves and do what they always wanted to do. As usual, there is probably a little of each side in every experience.

As nurses, we have met this often with patients and clients. Given a diagnosis of cancer, some people turn to the wall and give up, while others fight and even come to be thankful for a situation that can transform their lives. When we try to shield loved ones by 'not telling the truth', we may therefore deprive them of an opportunity to meet their deepest self.

The same applies to nurses – and indeed to many situations in life generally. It is only in moments of challenge that we come to know ourselves and our true values. What then happens is crucial, because we may suddenly find that we had values we never knew of, or that values which we expected to find simply seem not to be there. When we therefore make assumptions about people and how they will react to a challenge, we can be very surprised. Not only do patients find the vigour to fight an illness when they thought they had not an ounce of strength left, but nurses too find that they have powers they were not aware of and courage they never before met in themselves.

An image often used to describe such moments is that of the butterfly emerging from the chrysalis. A spectacularly beautiful creature emerges from a (usually) dull brown pupa. In much of nature, the offspring is recognisably the same, but in this case something so utterly different is produced that it takes a leap of the mind to imagine how a crawling caterpillar first changed itself into a static chrysalis and then emerged as a delicate flying object with every cell changed twice over.

As humans, we are bound by our physicality, but in character and attitude we can change from one state into another. Many people experience this as a midlife crisis, and the banker turned historian or the shop manager turned teacher should not surprise us. The retiring mother turned activist and 'the man whose hobby was to raise pedigree budgies, until he celebrated his retirement by opening all the cages and letting them all fly free' (Bruce, 1999, p. 108) will all have come to a moment when they truly 'found' themselves and, like the cucumber, became uncurved.

Damasio (1994) argues that Descartes' 'I think, therefore I am' is fundamentally wrong. He says that 'we are, and then we think' (p. 248). Because we are what we are, we can change how we think about this being. When we come to know ourselves truly, often through some unexpected challenge, we also become truly human. It is this potential for people to be and to become that we acknowledge when we say that people matter. Anything that might diminish this potential is essentially unethical and needs to be questioned.

Respect for persons

Oppenheimer (1995, p. 63) believes that the principle that 'people matter' is 'a great improvement upon "respect for persons"'. She believes that the expression 'people matter' is less formal, and therefore 'it is also less legalistic and potentially more comprehensive'. Oppenheimer is well aware of the possible pitfalls in making such a statement because who or what is a person has been argued for thousands of years and is even more sharply focused today when the life and death of patients are constantly a matter not only of caring, but also of financial consideration.

The debates about abortion and euthanasia are largely about the concept of person and personhood, and consequently the rights attached to such concepts. When life is described as 'sacred', this has usually been applied only to human life. This is fast changing, and we recognise a new sacredness in animals, trees and drops of water. To say that life is sacred is not adequate, but to respect only persons is not adequate either because we may need to respect water and air first as we cannot live without them. Oppenheimer has a strong point therefore when she says that people matter: it is a more specific term. And what she says with this term is that 'the mattering of people has everything to do with their capacity to *mind* and be *minded about*' (p. 63, original emphasis). She goes on to say that it might be possible to 'define a person as a "pattern of lovability"', a term that she borrows from Jenkins (1966, pp. 2–3). This may be both an emotive term and also one which might stretch the challenge of nursing into uncharted territories. All nurses have to care for all types of patient, some of whom are not lovable, or who are abusive, unresponsive, demanding or so ill that one wishes them dead. Having to care for such people is enough of a chore; loving them is too much. But this is not what is meant here. Someone being or having a 'pattern of lovability' means more an acknowledgement of that person as a person: such a person was once loved by a mother, a family, friends. He or she was in turn capable of loving others. This person has a name; this person matters, even now in circumstances that may be far from optimal.

Respect for persons is frequently described as an ethical principle. Churchill (1994, p. 328) says that the Golden Rule 'Do unto others as you would be done by' could be used 'to portray a world in which one's own self-regard and self-interest become yardsticks for imagining what the desires of another might be'. In this context, this means a reciprocity: each helping the other and each needing the other. In helping each other in our needs, we share one another's burdens and respond to and out of a pattern of lovability.

Here a nurse describes her relationship with a patient whom she had nursed some years before:

> She cried, of course she cried. We all cried with her. That is the sort of relationship we have with the patients. It can be very emotionally draining, but it is also very satisfying.

Unexpectedly meeting the patient again later when she had got a new job, the nurse said:

> When I met Julie in the day room after I'd got the job, we were hugging and laughing and she was as pleased for me as I was for myself. (Dobb and Small, 1997)

When nurses and patients can freely enjoy each other's company and enhance each other's well-being, surely they do this as persons rather than as functionaries in a role. Such moments are rare, however, and cannot be expected, but when they do happen, they last for a long time.

Perhaps one way in which we recognise another person's respect for us is in the look in the other's eye when we are congratulated or paid a compliment. How genuine is the look? Is the praise really meant, or is it given grudgingly? The 'moral artists' (see Chapter 9) are those people who are willing to express their beliefs in ways in which others can perceive and recognise their own experience. Nurses regularly act as moral artists. When we can share with our patients our own hurts and pains, joys and delights, we can paint or sculpt for them something to look at and perhaps measure their own imagination against. People matter, completely and utterly, and simply 'respecting persons' is perhaps no longer an adequate enough concept, although the ethical principle remains.

Individuals and society

Does the individual matter more, or does society? The language of rights has made us much more conscious of individual needs and wants. Because we have grown accustomed to this language and therefore to individualism, we have tended to neglect the counterbalancing need for responsibility and social justice. This may, however, be too simplistic a view and one which is also entirely dualistic. The idea that 'people matter' may be helpful here in understanding how individuals and society interact.

The UK and many other Western countries have long traditions of paternalistic regimes inherited from centuries of struggles to survive. Giving power to the state or classes of individuals – such as physicians – meant that individuals had no choice but to accept paternalism. The masses of the people therefore never needed to question their predicament or conditions. What one could not challenge, one might be better off accepting. Beauchamp and Childress (1989, p. 217), however, argue that 'the dominant reason why paternalism is unacceptable is that the rightful authority resides in the individual whose life is controlled, not in the controller'. By dint of being human, we are each at the same time controllers and controlled. We live in houses built by others and in states ruled by others. Even though we may have chosen the house we live in or the government that rules us, we have limited control once we have embarked on a major course.

In order to be and remain human, we have to exercise our creative abilities. This means at one level physical reproduction: creating other persons. At another level, it means teaching, educating, sharing and co-operating with other people: also creating other persons. The fact that we are born from another person makes us social beings. Our earliest life is entirely dependent on the relationship of the person who cares for us and her or his willingness to nurture us. The *milieu* in which we grow up shapes us long before we can question it.

'Nature' creates each person individually and uniquely. This individuality extends to the smallest visible items: even one snowflake is different from another. Only geneticists seem to have found the means of reproduction in nature that is entirely the same.

Oppenheimer (1995, p. 63) asks, 'if human beings seem to be given responsibility by their Creator to create other persons... how far does this responsibility extend?' This is a very useful question for nurses, who clearly often give of their own physical and emotional health and well-being in their care for others.

When AIDS first came on the scene, some nurses refused to care for patients, saying that they brought the illness upon themselves by their lifestyle and practices. If this view were extended, it could mean that nurses might refuse to care for patients with heart disease because they brought it upon themselves by smoking, diabetics for eating too much sugar, people with sports injuries because they engaged in dangerous pursuits, patients with colonic cancer for not eating enough roughage and asthmatics for breathing polluted air.

This does not take into account that many diseases and illnesses are caused by society. Poverty, inadequate housing and the destruction of neighbourhoods and communities by unemployment and the closure of industries are largely beyond the control of many people and are equally responsible for many diseases that may be preventable, given the right conditions. It is therefore unrealistic to blame one person for causing heart disease through smoking for enjoyment and not blaming another person whose heart disease has been caused through smoking that has become part of a culture of unemployment and disillusion.

Our culture is quick to condemn and often slow to tackle the real causes of ill health and vulnerability. It is here that nurses have an important ethical responsibility. Every patient and client whom we treat and meet needs to be treated and met not only as an individual, but also as an individual-in-society. It is not enough that we rescue the people about to drown: we have to confront the cause of the drowning. This is as much part of the treatment as is the actual care itself. It is here that nurses personally and nursing generally need to be much more active themselves, as well as being taken seriously in their preventive work.

Campbell (1997, p. 131) writes that:

in Western thought the value of the individual has often been given priority over membership of family, social group or nation. In medical ethics the principle of respect for autonomy may appear to favour individualism, but in medicine and in ethics the isolated individual is a misleading abstraction. We deserve respect as individuals, but our health and our moral choices require communal support and responsibility.

The support and responsibility given to people generally is in the first instance that they are listened to. In any conflict or dilemma, what matters is that individual stories can be told. This requires that they are heard. Too often, however, we see only a crisis and a need to fix it, be it with medical interventions or convoys of food. The further away from the actual situation we are, the more detached our actions become and the more society orientated our views.

It is easy to argue that, when we are concerned with individuals, we become 'involved' and therefore lose objectivity. When we are caring and supporting other people, we give them the opportunity to tell their stories. The responsibility is in the act of listening. Clearly, an individual story cannot be applied to a group of people, however small or however similar, but it is the individual story that highlights aspects of the wider story. The Hastings Center Report (1998, p. 28) describes a case study of an elderly woman with a history of emphysema and manic depression admitted for shortness of breath. She had no relatives but two friends, and had written an advance directive some years previously. After first acute and then long-term treatment, she seemed content to spend her days watching television, presumably unable to make decisions regarding her care. Her friends asked that the living will be activated. The nursing staff and attending physician argued against this, but an ethics committee finally agreed, and she was transferred to another hospital where her life support was disconnected and she died a few days later.

This is perhaps not an everyday story in Britain, but it is a reminder of how decisions by committee see the legal aspects of a situation and the teleological consequences for society. Indeed, it may be right that the law regarding advance directives needs to be strengthened or refined, as does the power of committees. What one also needs to see in this case is that the caring personnel were listened to but not heard, consulted but not regarded. I venture to guess that the committee (subconsciously) feared the power of the caring staff and that the staff (subconsciously) feared their own power. This leads to the argument that much of what goes on in medicine is not an ethical problem *as such* but is a problem of power between the various professions involved in care. Nurses can and need to address this by taking their power seriously. It is in their care for individuals that they can make their message – that they matter – heard in society. It is the individual person who matters but the individual-in-society who counts.

Holistic relationships

There will always be a tension between the needs, rights and wants of the individual and those of society. This is the creative tension that matters – people matter – and we have to discover constantly anew how we use this tension.

When people are ill or have had an accident, they gain by this a reason for telling their story. A new meaning for their existence has presented itself, and they make sense of this situation by telling their story. Our culture, however, has succeeded in largely suppressing this need. Tests and machines now make a diagnosis based on norms, and interventions have replaced the long stays in bed when the body could often find its own level of healing. Our technological culture has deprived us in many ways of the content for telling our stories (Mordacci and Sobel, 1998, p. 36) and hence of the relationships that lead to wholeness. It is therefore all the more important that we re-affirm that people – not just our technology – matter and that this can only happen when we listen to their stories and make sure that our own stories are heard.

The feminist literature in particular sheds new light on the whole area of relationships. Noddings (1984, p. 2) describes the feminine 'voice' as being 'rooted in receptivity, relatedness, and responsiveness'. Through caring, she says, women are in a special relationship with others that 'provides the motivation for us to be moral' (p. 5).

Those who are involved in the daily care of people create relationships, and such relationships are and become the vital elements in life. Mordacci and Sobel (1998, pp. 36–7) describe the various aspects that define 'health', mentioning in particular 'pathogens' and 'salutogens'. 'Pathogenic factors may be biological, genetic, family related, social, economic, educational or environmental. Pathogenic viruses, or bacteria, a diet high in saturated fat, smoking, excessive alcohol, a defective immune system cause maladies that disable individuals.' These, the authors say, can be treated or prevented by physicians. What they call 'salutogens' are factors that enhance and produce health, such as freedom of choice, having one's basic needs met, 'curiosity, optimism, adaptability, a sense of humour, the capacity to love and to establish a durable intimate relationship with a fellow creature, whether human being or animal. Few, if any of the salutogenic factors have anything directly to do with medicine or physicians.'

If these factors have little to do with medicine or physicians, they certainly have to do with nursing. Nursing relies first and foremost on the relationship between nurse and patient. Most people regard all those who concern themselves with their health and illness as important. They touch them – unlike bankers, shop assistants and the many other people on whom we depend. 'Touch is closely interwoven with identity, with survival, with the cultural signs of sex, status and aggression; all this makes touch the most immediate, most intimate and most commanding form of human communication' (Routasalo, 1997, p. 7). Nursing *care* almost always involves touch, and this immediately establishes (or not) an intimate relationship. Such relationships can only be holistic when 'curiosity, optimism, [and] adaptability' are present in a direction from the nurse to the patient. If the patient is temporarily not able to respond in the same way, it is again the kind of relationship which the nurse has that can foster this and empower the patient.

Holistic relationships are also 'salutogenic' in the sense that they contribute to health more essentially than we often are aware of. Would it not be possible to imagine that the nurses in the case described above were 'salutogenic' for the patient, enabling for her a kind a life that had some purpose, even if it were a very restricted one?

The following story was told me by a nurse. It has been slightly adapted to maintain confidentiality.

> A teenager had presented himself to a school nurse with cuts, saying that he had fallen off his bicycle and cut himself on some sharp edges of torn metal. While the nurse dressed his wounds he volunteered to her that in fact he had been in a fight and that he had a knife on him. The nurse knew this boy's family from a previous employment, and there and then made a deal with him. She was legally under an obligation to report the incident not only to the head teacher, but also to the police, but she was prepared to take a risk. She told the teenager that she would keep the knife and not make any report if he agreed to see her once a week for counselling. He agreed and the two met regularly for some months. When both were satisfied that progress had been made, the nurse gave the knife to the young man and he handed it in at a police station. Later on he told her that the trust she had shown him had taught him more than many years of schooling.

Holistic relationships have far-reaching consequences. They depend on the circumstances, the people and the actions involved. Not everyone is asked to take risks of the kind that this nurse took, but any relationship involves risks; indeed, acting ethically will always involve risks. The boy was marked by this nurse's care, and she herself 'grew' as a person. This is the outcome: in giving we receive. Holistic relationships are always two way.

Oppenheimer (1992, p. 47) says that 'roughly speaking, morality is about what ought to be done or not done, law is about what people can be compelled to do or not do'. In this case, it is possible to say that the nurse went beyond what she 'ought' to have done. Not only did she go beyond the call of duty, but she also acted entirely compassionately and altruistically. My guess is that, despite this, she will have had at least one sleepless night.

Story telling

We can only assert that people matter because we have been touched by their stories. The personal stories of individuals and the collective stories of families, groups and nations have formed us. Most of all, however, we are formed ourselves in the telling of our own story. The proverb 'I don't know what I think until I say it' is more realistic than might be implied. It is in our *ex*pression that we understand the *im*pression we have and make.

Story telling has become important in nursing, and much learning is achieved very fruitfully in this way. Telling the story is not enough, though. Listening to a story is important, but hearing it is crucial. 'I have never met a nurse who does not have a story to tell. Each story may have different facts and moral concerns, but every nurse lives with a case... etched into his or her memory' (Parker, 1990). Nurses learn a great deal from telling their stories in groups, comparing patients' and clients' diagnoses, treatments, outcomes and reactions. Stories and narratives are the basis for any organisation and profession to learn and maintain its identity, but this is not the only reason why stories are told. We tell each other stories because they have affected us, for better or for worse. It may be that there was an unusual diagnosis or illness, but more important is why this was perceived as unusual by the nurse who told the story. What made the nurse tell the story?

It is in telling our story that we define ourselves and are defined by others. Many of our stories are about events, other people and issues. As a counsellor, I listen to many stories, and my most crucial task is often to help clients to speak as themselves and start sentences with 'I', because we have learned that to speak in the neutral 'one' or 'you' gives us protection and distance, and is therefore safe. This is clearly necessary in many instances but not when it matters in human terms. Many of our stories are told in 'code' in order to make them acceptable to the listener in anticipation of what the reply might be. When we therefore tell stories in the first person, we take more risks with our lives, and this presumes a relationship based on trust. The relationship is therefore based on the shared stories as much as the stories themselves creating the relationship.

Every story is unique, and every story changes in the telling and to whom we tell it. It does not matter how well or inadequately the story is told; what matters, both for the person who tells it and for the person who hears it, is what is heard. It is because of this necessary interaction and time spent together that we assert that people matter.

The individual stories also become the larger story. A single patient's story becomes that of people with a similar disease, or background, or experience. A single nurse's story becomes that of a team, or a country, or the profession at large. We have to listen to each other's stories because patients are also citizens and nurses are also patients. The theme of this book is, however, that the nurses' story needs to be told more and heard more clearly. It therefore needs to be told more with that 'I' in front of it, and it has to be spoken and really heard rather than just listened to. It can only achieve this when nursing has heard well enough what the patients' story is. This means the stories of individuals, but also the stories of groups, nations and cultures. Nursing has to listen more globally more thoroughly and then tell its story and make sure that it is heard.

In telling each other our stories, we hear ourselves and understand ourselves. This is the therapeutic use of story telling. Those who educate nurses may say that this is not their domain: they are here to impart knowledge rather than to sort out mixed-up youngsters. But those very youngsters are asked to give holistic care, and that means taking every aspect of a person into consideration. When the body is diseased, the heart, the soul and the mind are just as much affected. When we know this but disregard it, we diminish not only another person, but also ourselves. We cannot say that 'people matter' and by that mean 'other people'. The other person's story is ultimately 'Everyman's' story. In order to be people who act ethically, we have to hear our own story first, thus establishing a set of criteria against which we can measure other stories.

Story telling also reflects the emotional fabric of caring. In nursing, where research is essentially about caring, it seems therefore incongruous that much of the academic language used in research is of an emotionally bare type. Surely it makes little sense, to research caring activities and then describe these in language where 'it is noted' or 'the author' writes as from a vantage point of untouched observer. Compassion demands also a language 'with passion'. Perhaps our academic institutions might be encouraged to pay more attention to how the research carried out by nursing students of all grades is written in order to reflect more adequately the emotional content in the academic context. It is difficult to foster the humanity of nurses in their work when academic work and printed material reflect the opposite.

In story telling it matters crucially what we listen *for*. If we tell stories of nursing diabetic patients in order to understand the diagnosis of diabetes, we listen for aspects of hyperglycaemia and hypoglycaemia. When we listen to a person, we hear something very different. Too often, however, we choose not to hear the other and we hear only ourselves, our own needs and what we want to hear. The 'I' needs to be given its rightful place.

In order to hear the real story, we have to train our ears to hear in a different way. Parker (1990, pp. 31–5) tells of the story of a patient who had had a stroke, having lost sensation and movement in his right side, and had difficulty in speaking and comprehending written and spoken words. When he had to undergo major surgery and painful dressing changes afterwards, the personnel caring for the patient considered the principle of the sanctity of life, constantly encouraging the patient to tolerate just a little more pain as this would help him to get better. This is taking a narrow view, applying one principle to the exclusion of alternative possibilities. This is also the point that Oppenheimer (1995, p. 63) makes by saying that 'respect for life' is not enough. In this instance, the nurses heard their own story by applying the principle of the sanctity of life indiscriminately. They did not see that their patient (the person) mattered more than a principle. Principles can very easily be seen as final arbiters and something absolute. Very little in life, however, is absolute. What we see may depend more on our vantage-point than on any absolute truth. Principles can guide us, but they also have to be set aside when we hear a person's cry for meaning. This is what story telling is generally about.

Receptivity

Among the aspects of relationships that Noddings (1984) mentions, receptivity has perhaps had least attention; relatedness and responsiveness have more currency. With receptivity, we receive something into ourselves. The basis of sharing starts here.

One aspect of 'people matter' is that we can truly affirm that people matter from experience rather than merely intellectually. This presupposes that we are willing to listen to each other's stories and be changed by what we hear. The stories may be of events or of memories, but every story told is a search for meaning and an attempt to make sense of an experience (Crawford *et al.*, 1992, p. 9).

When we tell our story to another person, we do so in order to hear ourselves and understand ourselves better. For that, we need the other person's response. It is not enough that we give an empathic response; empathy is 'a way of being' (Rogers, 1980, p. 143). Rogers might be describing receptivity when he says that 'to be with another in this way means that for the time being, you lay aside your own views and values in order to enter another's world without prejudice'. When this happens, the other person is indeed 'received' and affirmed. Without words, we convey that the other person matters. When we listen to the story, we are with that person in body and in mind. The 'echo' that we provide is not simply a repetition of the actual words spoken, but the words are amplified, the sound is fuller and it returns with a lapse of time, perhaps being repeated several times over. This is the empathic aspect of receptivity.

When listening to a story, we hear the whole person: the words chosen, the look in the eyes, the body language. We need to take all this in, and out of this complexity we respond.

Receptivity is a particularly feminine aspect of the psyche. However, this is not just women's domain but comprises the feminine part of caring that men as much as women possess. Rogers himself was a particularly good example of it in the way in which he listened to people.

Receptivity here means the listening part of a story telling situation. The one who tells the story is, however, also receptive as in real sharing there is no division into teller and listener, giver and receiver. Both have to tell and listen, give and take. Only in this way can dialogue be established and the story become useful, 'people matter' thus becoming a reality.

Receptivity relates to intuition. Noddings (1984, p. 162) says that 'to intuit the other' is also to receive the other. Noddings gives a whole list (p. 163) of how intuition has been understood and described in literature, for example as a source of truth, as a special tool with which to understand life, as art, as the source of moral judgement and as connecting reason and experience. When caring for others, we know the direction in which to go, but we must constantly be open to new developments, and these may be supplied by intuition.

Being receptive means being open to new ideas and experiences. It is a willingness to be challenged and changed by people, events and objects. There is in that a childlike curiosity and delight that is part of the trust which is necessary in affirming that 'people matter'.

Relatedness

The world over, people cry and laugh for similar reasons; that alone relates us to every other human being. We may not all laugh at the same jokes or hold the same values, but love, fear, joy and anger are universally recognisable.

In nursing, there is an immediate relatedness with nurses everywhere. We recognise a similarity and bond in the work we do. As nurses we also recognise an instinct to help when we see someone ill or injured or in some other need that we can fulfil. There is a relatedness between human need and human skill at every level. When we see someone in need, that person's need calls forth in us a response. We do not first ask how much it will cost in terms of effort or involvement, but we respond because in a way we recognise our own need reflected in the other.

It is almost impossible, when considering relatedness, not to mention Buber's (1937) *I and Thou*. We relate to others as Thou when we relate to them truly, but it is only in relation that we can say 'Thou'. Everything else, Buber contends, is an I–It relation, as with objects. It would be difficult to relate to a washing machine in the same way as to a person, even though we use the washing machine frequently and depend on it. Yet for many people, their relationship with their computer is more I–Thou than I–It, especially when it exasperates them. Equally, some personal relationships can be demeaning rather than enhancing; one need only think of that between hostage taker and hostage. We tend to think that only in very intimate relationships do we address the other as Thou, but the point that Buber makes is that all personal relationships have aspects of I–Thou. We can only address another person as Thou when we are deeply convinced that people matter, and conversely, when we do affirm this, every other human being has the character of Thou.

If we say that people matter, they matter in the sense that our relationships with them are to be humanising and creative. In the way in which we respond to people lies the clue to how to do it.

Nurses want to care for others and are conditioned early on that if they cannot cope emotionally with such care, nursing is not for them. Hence we have the big problem of nurses finding it difficult to care for each other and being cared for. Ideas of self-sacrifice, although rarely called such or admitted to, are embedded in the nursing culture and can too easily be exploited. The I–Thou relationship can then deteriorate into I–It, and when this happens, we see the other person only as a means to an end rather than an end in her- or himself. When this happens, we need to ask where not only our ethics but also our vision and our reason for being in a caring profession, have gone.

We can only truly say 'Thou' to another person when we have learned truly to say 'I'. This means 'I' with all the positive and negative aspects of the personality. For most people, this is a life's work and is not easily achieved. Perhaps it is possible to say that while individual nurses are learning such insights more readily, nursing as a profession is still on the threshold of such a belief and practice.

Buber understood 'Thou' to be both the other person and also that which is bigger than ourselves: the transcendent Other: God. One leads to the other, but in each instance, we need the balance of the 'I'. When we have clearer notions of what we mean by each aspect, we recognise that the use of 'I' and 'Thou' is the use of a power. How we use our power is significant. Every time we say 'Thou', we give away our power and empower the other. When this happens, the other can say 'Thou' to us and so empower us. The use of power is shared, unlike the situations when paternalism is the rule of the game. When we say that 'people matter', we touch on this idea of empowering ourselves by empowering others.

It is possible to say that all ethics is about power and the use of power. This is clearly seen in the following quote from Kuhse (1997, pp. 199–200):

> What [is] significant from the nurses' point of view [is] not only the substantive question of whether the doctors' actions [are] right or wrong, but also the implicit assumption that it is appropriate for doctors to make morally significant end-of-life decisions and for nurses to carry them out (or at least to consent to them) regardless of their own moral or professional point of view. These cases signal that nurses are not regarded as autonomous health-care professionals and moral agents, but as dependent functionaries whose role it is to do the moral bidding of others.

This single extract points to the various topics addressed in this chapter. When other people are not treated as morally equal, they are not respected, not addressed as Thou; the relationship with them is not considered to be as important; their actions are downgraded and their opinions dismissed; and one's own power is abused and that of others not considered as mattering. In short, 'people matter' is not something that is applied in this instance.

Kuhse (1997, p. 216) pleads for *systemic* (original emphasis) change. I can only echo her call, but I am saying that, unless nurses recognise their own strength, they cannot make such systemic change. By outlining some of the points, especially from the domain of ethics, by which such strength can be gained, I hope that such systemic change can come about. One of the needs to consider particularly is that of the relationships and the kind of powers that are at work in them.

Responsiveness

In the context of a nurse–patient relationship, responsiveness means:

a willingness to accept a patient's invitation to be a close travelling companion on an uncertain journey. Experiences of intense pain, abandonment, and fear of living and dying are shared in an effort to co-construct the meaning of seemingly meaningless experiences. (Parker, 1990, p. 38)

Parker goes on to say that this 'necessitates engaged listening, authentic responsiveness, mutual disclosure, and negotiation'.

Responding to people, events and ideas is what makes and keeps us human. There is nothing so beautiful as a baby's first smile, signifying a first responsiveness. Most nurses will also know the thrill of getting a sign, however small, from an unconscious patient, recognising in that a first return to some form of consciousness. Relating to such a responsive person is different from relating to an unconscious person.

A conversation is a series of responses in which each person interprets what the other has said and answers in the light of a process of weighing up memories and possible outcomes of what is being said. Most of the time, we are barely aware of this process. We sometimes say something inspired or something that we regret, and we cannot think why we said it. The other person responds, and in the further unfolding of the conversation, the responses make the relationship grow or diminish.

Clearly, we respond not only to words, but also to the whole situation in which we find ourselves. As we respond, so we are responded to. Our ability to respond leads to the recognition of our responsibility. To walk by on the other side when we see someone in need and we can help diminishes us as persons; it diminishes our 'I'. In terms of the stories we tell each other, we need to be receptive and hear the whole story, in particular the story that is actually told rather than that which we want to hear. We relate to the other person in the way that is most fitting: not with the ears of rules, regulations or principles, but with the ears of knowledge that people matter. This is far more liberating – and often also more daring and loving – than any theory, however perfect.

Our personal power lies in our responsibility. The power is shared and it is therefore real power, not abused power. Power has rightly been seen to be corrupting. One way of making

use of power positively is in acknowledging that p
not only I, me and myself, but 'I and Thou'.

The fact, then, that 'people matter' is so basic t
and to living in general – that it must be seen as
guides us in everything that we undertake. We act m
ethically when we act as if people matter. It is from that basis
that we can and must assert that nurses matter.

3

Mattering Matters

Nursing works from the basic premise that people are important. At the same time, nursing asserts that the members of its profession are important as people and as individuals. Because people matter, nurses matter. This gives nursing as a profession strength in its collective vision and gives individual nurses the right and the duty to make their voices heard. In this chapter, I will be looking more specifically at what this implies for nurses. The term 'mattering matters' needs, however, to be clarified first in the way in which Oppenheimer uses it.

Mattering matters

Oppenheimer (1995, p. 65) calls the term 'mattering' 'a bridge between fact and value'. She also uses the term 'minding' in the same way. 'People matter because they mind.'

Whenever the term 'mind' is used, we are in danger of falling into any number of traps that have tried to describe what is meant. Oppenheimer does not dismiss the vast array of literature on the subject, but she is concerned with using language that is more acceptable in a world where dualistic concepts are no longer adequate. She makes clear that a person does not consist of two entities: a body and a mind; instead, a person consists of all the entities together. Oppenheimer says:

> A person is not two beings, one conscious, the other physical. We have after all come across enough people to recognise what they are. A person just is this double kind of being... Yet surely bodies and souls are still distinct notions? By all means: something can be derivative without being unreal. This is a matter of organising our ideas, not of denying any of them. (Oppenheimer, 1988, p. 45)

Once it is clear that mind is not just a mental activity, but that minds need bodies, it is difficult to be abstract about the concept of mind. Any idea of wholeness – especially in health care – must include all aspects of the person rather than just a disease or a diagnosis. Thus, Oppenheimer (1995, p. 65) says that 'to progress from minding as mental activity to minding as caring, and then from caring to loving, is not to slither down a slippery slope but to develop understanding'. Her conclusion is that 'embodied minds – that is, people – *mind* in the richer sense, and therefore *matter*'.

Mattering as the bridge between fact and value

The 'fact' that Oppenheimer sees as needing a bridge is a legacy of a philosophical taking-to-pieces that has left us with detachment, moralism and 'a great deal [of] duty and not much about what makes life worth living' (1995, p. 64). Morality is not something abstract, and duty is not something that can be dissected, but this is what has happened in the West, at least since the time of Descartes. Our whole society has been shaped by the belief that:

> reason is a natural disposition of the human mind, which when governed by proper education can discover certain truths

and the assumption:

> that the clarity and distinctness of these truths or the veracity of their impact upon our senses would be sufficient to ensure inter-subjective agreement among like thinking rational minds. (Benhabib, 1992, p. 4)

We cannot undo our past or deny our heritage, but we do not need to perpetuate thought patterns and ideas if they are either no longer applicable today or indeed hinder our endeavour.

The values that we deduce from these facts have governed our moral and ethical behaviour, but they too are now questionable. Oppenheimer (1995, pp. 64–5) concludes that 'ethical discussion tended to arrive soon at questions about what people could be blamed for doing or not doing. Anything beyond duty was supererogation, not generosity. It seemed naïve to mention "love"'.

The bridge that 'mattering' creates is that it unites a reasoning about duties and the possibility that we can love patients and use those words with integrity. Oppenheimer, being a philosopher, argues more subtly and in more detail, but, by using her terms, I hope to show that the concept can translate into practical spheres within and for nursing.

Our thoughts matter

If nursing is to make an impact in the future of health care both nationally and globally, it matters not only what we think, but also that our thoughts can be translated into action. This is a daily dilemma for many nurses. Cavill (1998, p. 22) asks 'why, when they have so much to offer, nurses are not heard and are left feeling frustrated' below a cartoon in which two nurses discuss a document entitled 'Ethical Dilemmas' as some doctors walk into the ward. The caption from one of the nurses is 'Should I tell the consultant what I really think of him?' This is only the tip of an iceberg of much thinking that is never voiced because nurses are generally not taken seriously.

Nurses are not involved in much decision making because they are never asked, and also because they have never spoken their thoughts. There is a strong sense that we are worth less and therefore what we think is less important. This comes from the time when women were considered inferior and when reason reigned supreme. Today's ethical problem is no longer that we do our duty and obey but that people matter, and therefore their thoughts matter – whoever the people are. Other people, for example doctors and politicians, have to listen as part of their duty, but nurses have to speak their thoughts as part of their ethical duty. It *ought* to matter and therefore it does, and we *should* mind that we have this duty and responsibility, and we need to take it. What we 'mind' about 'matters' to us.

Nolan (1996, p. 1030) describes how, in his first ever lecture, he said that that bathing patients was a basic nursing task. This was interpreted as meaning unimportant and of little interest. Nolan had to rely on 'a well known member of the profession' to come to his rescue and point out that he had surely meant the word in the sense of 'fundamental' or 'essential'. He describes feeling inadequate at getting his message across and being surprised that it was misinterpreted. We have all found ourselves in similar situations, but not all of us have had the benefit of a senior person's help and interpretation.

This little incident points to one of the crucial elements of why the thoughts of nurses are not heard and therefore often not spoken: language and assumptions. Because we have not learned well enough to express ourselves unambiguously or to stay to make a point, those listening are making assumptions about what we mean. When we realise what has happened, we have to rely on others to put us right. It then takes a person of integrity and empathy to interpret correctly and not take advantage of the other person's faltering. I believe that it is largely a fact of inculturation that nurses have 'unlearned' how to speak clearly and make their point with deliberation. This happens in individual situations, and these may be isolated, but the general culture of nursing has the mindset that makes such stereotypes sadly still a fact. Nurses generally may be quite vocal and accepted, but nursing as a profession suffers from a deep sense of being sidelined and diminished. Indeed, nurses seem to glory from such behaviour. In an article entitled 'The long and winding road', Hancock (1998, p. 24) describes the positive aspects of the White Paper on the health services published in 1997. The tone of her paper is optimistic and positive, acknowledging that nurses are at last taken seriously by policy makers. She ends by saying that 'nurses have had to travel a long road to get recognition for the work they do – and the journey is not over yet'. A cartoon taking a large space of the article shows two nurses, one of them saying, 'So when I said we don't get the recognition we deserve he said "er, who are you?"' Despite the up-beat tone of the article, the cartoon and the title of the article demonstrate the culture of self-punishment and under-valuing all too well, reinforcing the negative image of nursing.

Snee and Salter (1997, p. 40) bluntly say that 'nursing has confused the cosmetic appearance of professional status with the reality of occupational power in the health service'. They believe that much has been achieved in terms of higher education-based training, clinical grading structure and a pay review body, but, in terms of power, nothing much has changed. If anything has changed, it has been from nursing to management. The future should be a more sophisticated approach by nursing:

> Unfortunately, if understandably, the reaction to this has produced a mind-set that tends to withdraw into the occupational enclave, limit engagement with other occupational groups and protect the purity of the nursing identity. Such isolationism – reinforced by the supposed acquisition of professional autonomy – has allowed others to define the occupational agenda for the health service as a whole. Purity is only of symbolic value if power has been lost. (Snee and Salter, 1997, p. 41)

It is this possibility that others will define the occupational agenda for nurses, which should be the driving force. In Oppenheimer's words, we should 'mind' about that. This means not only that our thoughts and minds are exercised, but also that the whole of our being, feelings and actions are included. Because we mind – passionately, absolutely – it matters. I believe that we need to show the world much more thoroughly that we do indeed mind, by making our thinking much clearer.

Garbett (1997, p. 41) describes how the Royal College of Nursing (RCN) is advocating evidence-based practice (a trend drawn from medicine) in its Institute, the RCNI. This is a merger of the former Institute of Advanced Nursing Education, the Daphne Heald Research Unit in London and the National Institute for Nursing in Oxford. The RCNI gained joint fourth place in a Research Assessment Exercise covering 36 institutions carried out in 1996. Alison Kitson, the RCNI's director, is quoted as saying that:

> perhaps the reason why nursing has not felt entitled to join the evidence-based movement is that in its current stage of development it is still at the stage of knowledge generation. We still need a lot of investment to *describe properly* what it is that we do. (emphasis added)

This reinforces what I have been describing as the mountain of experience (Chapter 1). We need to describe this mountain not just to ourselves, but also to the world at large.

Our feelings matter

The feelings that nursing engenders must be taken seriously: first by nurses as an important, valid and guiding element of our work; and second by politicians of all kinds, who may dismiss them as a dispensable byproduct of a job. So that they can get the 'feel' for the importance of feelings, we need to express far more clearly what is at stake: the health of every person's integrity. Oppenheimer (1995, pp. 65–6) muses that:

> the literal meaning of 'mattering' is 'having substance'. Something which 'doesn't matter' has no substance, no weight.

In this way, the literal and the metaphorical are understood as the same.

> Likewise the meanings of 'minding'... run into each other. One plain meaning of 'minding' is 'attending'. Attention seems neutral and value-free: but is it?... Can you imagine a 'mind', however elementary, which attended but did not care?

In this way, facts and values are bridged by 'minding' and 'mattering'. Attending and caring involve much thinking and feeling.

That our feelings are important at all levels is not often disputed among practising nurses. It is only as we get further and further away from actual care that we become suspicious and fearful of feelings and try to 'shield' practitioners with policies and instructions. Nurses recognise this clearly enough but, as so often, may not be able to say exactly what it is they recognise when they see legislation driving a wedge between them and their care.

The feelings that matter in nursing are often hard to describe. What is involved? In a series of 'Nursing narratives' published in Nursing Times in 1992 and 1993, many 'feelings' were mentioned, often without being labelled or defined. A nurse caring for Roy, a man with learning disabilities, recalls:

> I know I have made a difference in his life, but it is not something that can be measured. The difference lies in our friendship, based on equality and mutual respect. We give each other something special. I know it and he does, too. (Anonymous, 1993, p. 42)

I have found other people's tears hard to cope with in the past, and had usually pretended not to notice them. But this time the absolute misery I saw in front of me completely knocked aside my embarrassment. ...I finally understood what 'being with' a patient meant. I had been frightened to allow people to cry because I felt inadequate. (Shepherdson, 1992, p. 35)

As we looked at each other I felt that no matter what I said to this man, it would be trivial, as he lay fighting for his life. I told him slowly that I did not know what to say to him, and with that he took my hand that had been resting on the bed and enclosed it in his own two, and closed his eyes. We stayed like that for the remainder of time I was with him – each drawing strength from the contact we had with each other. Before I returned to the ward I said goodbye, and thanked him. (Summers, 1992, p. 47)

These stories describe the feelings that nurses encounter in contact with patients, and they are the substance of job satisfaction. They are the reasons for many nurses to stay in work when other pressures might push them into leaving. Sharing such feelings with colleagues can be the basis for support and education, constituting role modelling and therefore being essential to the building-up of the corpus of nursing knowledge.

Yet there are also the feelings that represent the opposite spectrum: feelings of anger, resentment, impotence, worthlessness and guilt. These feelings drive us just as much as do the gentler and more positive ones.

Stories of nurses being ridiculed in front of patients (Mort, 1996, p. 40) and having their concerns disregarded (Anonymous, 1998a, p. 35) or their views dismissed as unimportant (RCN, undated) ought to make us see red. Such incidences clearly show that people do not matter to those concerned, in particular that nurses do not matter. It is possible to make allowances and excuses, but there is a limit to such generosity. It is impossible to be belittled and not be affected by this. When one kind of feeling is activated, others almost always follow and this can only be destructive. It is a strong person who can pick herself up and get on with 'normal' life.

In 1986, Collière noted that women are rendered 'invisible' by systems of care that are driven by economic forces. Having become 'invisible', Collière (1986, p. 106) describes women as 'having lost their own references and the ability to use them properly and feeling they might do wrong, they develop a sense of guilt, show no self-confidence and therefore build up a very poor image of themselves'. When feelings such as these are disregarded, they become destructive for individuals and society. It is for this reason, if for no other, that they need to be taken seriously: they matter.

Acting in accordance with one's ethical reasoning and feelings has been studied by Åström *et al.* (1993, p. 179). These Swedish researchers found that, in many situations experienced, nurses were aware of either loneliness or togetherness. The language used when relating their care episodes led to further divisions into whether situations were overwhelming or possible to grasp. The researchers found that, in situations possible to grasp, the nurses used terms such as 'I' and 'we' when referring to themselves and their co-actors, but in overwhelming situations, terms such as 'one' and 'they' were more common. Those nurses who had support groups coped more easily, but those who had no such groups 'reported difficulties acting in accordance with their ethical reasoning and feelings'. Perhaps this seems an obvious conclusion, but it must add to the knowledge base and the need to voice and externalise why nurses act in the way they do.

It is sometimes clearly necessary to be taken to the limit before we do something about it. Only then do we have enough energy to act. Maybe there are those who exploit the lethargy of nurses, taking it for granted – or so they think – that nurses will not put up a fight. The 'divide-and-rule' tactic is very subtle. In today's health care system where resources are increasingly scarce, many nurses prefer to keep their heads down. But it does matter that they mind. This is perhaps the really important focus on feelings. The 'longing for goodness' is there at every stage, and the need to express this is perhaps one of the strongest driving forces.

Our commitment matters

Kocher (1997, p. 64) describes how the annual congress of the Swiss Nurses Association tried to make sense of the theme 'The hidden face of care', making the invisible visible. She says that:

many people prove their commitment and enormous professionalism in this work [of clarifying, explaining, measuring and classi-
fying] which is certainly going to be fruitful and will advance nursing
as an autonomous activity. But no classification, however sophisticated, can measure what happens in a human relationship, in its
richness and intensity, because this remains invisible. ...but we must
not forget that this mystery is an integral part of the act of caring.
(translated by current author)

It is not that personal and professional commitment is lacking.
Instead, the commitment shown by many nurses is either taken
for granted or seen as dangerous. Chambliss (1996, p. 67)
says that:

caring requires a personal commitment of the nurse to her work.
It requires a commitment of the nurse herself, as a person, to her
work. There is an intertwining of professional skills and personal
involvement; in a sense, the involvement is the work, in a way not
true of more technical occupations.

The stories above of the three nurses who describe their feelings also show their commitment. The personal involvement
means that much is given and also that much is received in return.

A definition of 'commitment' has been attempted by Roach
(1992, p. 65) when she says that 'commitment is... a complex
affective response characterized by a convergence between one's
desires and one's obligations, and by a deliberate choice to act
in accordance with them'. Roach sees commitment as one of
the five elements that constitute caring (along with compassion, competence, confidence and conscience). She says that:

devotion (commitment) is essential in caring: if devotion (commitment) breaks down, caring breaks down. Therefore, commitment
is a quality of investment of self in a task, a person, a choice, or
a career, a quality which becomes so internalized as a value that
what I am obligated to do is not regarded as a burden. Rather, it
is a call which draws me to a conscious, willing and positive course
of action.

Commitment is one of those things which is not much thought
about until it is questioned. Why do we remain committed to
a particular patient, job or cause? Clearly, what we get from
staying with people or institutions determines how much we
are willing to give in return. When the give-and-take is more

or less equal, there is no problem, but when this balance becomes distorted, an adjustment of values takes place.

It is impossible to describe, measure or pay for the commitment that nurses give. The schedules of unsocial hours, risks of contamination and injuries, abuse suffered from frightened or mischievous persons, and sheer weight of responsibility for the welfare of people who are ill and dependent cannot simply be taken for granted by society in general and employers and politicians in particular. It can be discussed in the classroom, but it cannot be taught as a subject. Yet, unless commitment is there, as Roach (1992, p. 65) points out, what care is given is not given caringly.

In her theory of human caring, Watson (1994, p. 3) emphasises that 'caring is the heart of nursing and the ethical and philosophical foundation for our acts'. She is clear that the *being* and *knowing* of caring are 'related to caring-healing relationships and practices [which] are critical to health and quality of living'. Her colleague Nyberg (1994, p. 56) believes that commitment can be taught to nurses by:

> treating them like professionals and expecting them to commit to their patients throughout their health or illness episode. ...Patient assignment should be made so that one nurse takes care of a patient repeatedly.

What these authors are pointing to is that the commitment in nursing is not something that is taught in front of a class, prescribed or expected, but something which is shared. The act of treating nurses professionally – as if they mattered – assures that they can commit themselves. This simply reinforces the thesis that people matter. When we acknowledge each other as people with full potential, we can and will use that potential. When we see a person, we see also what concerns that person; the person matters and what she or he minds about matters: mattering matters. Sharing ourselves first enables others also to share.

It matters that nurses are committed, and what they commit themselves to matters. In instances in the literature too numerous to mention, it is pointed out again and again that when nurses are given responsibility and are consulted on matters that affect them both directly and indirectly, they are more able and willing to use their talents to the full. On the other hand, when decisions are made concerning them but without consulting them, they become disillusioned. Morale drops, individuals become unwilling to respond productively to changes or threats and an insensitivity to outside forces grows, leading to introspection (Castledine, 1997a, p. 773). Many forces have enormous power over nurses, often making individual nurses prone to feeling no better than a cog in a vast machine. These same forces also have the power to do the opposite. It is not necessarily more pay, but being treated as a professional, that represents the 'feel-good factor'. When one health authority tried to do this in the spring of 1998 by giving each nurse a Mars bar, however, this was rightly perceived to be an insult rather than a homage.

Every nurse knows what her or his commitment is, or was, or could be. It is not simply an ideal but a fact of life that is part of why we want to be nurses. In Nyberg's (1994, p. 56) description of what constitutes the process of caring, 'self-worth' is placed first. She says that 'nurses must learn to appreciate their own self and attend to their own needs to learn and grow'. It is this basic attitude that is able to affirm 'I'm OK', which is vital if we are to make the message clear that what we do as nurses matters. However, even phrases such as 'nurses must learn' point to the future, to something that will come. The fact is that nurses already know and believe that they matter. Our commitment *now* is crucial, and it is crucial that we work with what is there, because that is what we know.

Our knowledge matters

The knowledge that nurses have both individually and as a profession is phenomenal. Much of it is underused or dormant:

> By identifying gaps in services and suggesting possible solutions, nurses are... best placed to ensure that these developments are patient-focused. (Sams, 1998, p. 77)

The first of the following quotes outlines the definition of the American Nurses Association of a clinical nurse specialist:

a nurse with clinical experience in a specialized area of nursing who provides leadership for the development of nursing practice through a variety of activities such as staff development, education, consultation and research as well as direct patient care. (Briody, 1996, p. 17)

Six of the eight nurse-led pilots given the go-ahead under the NHS (Primary Care) Act, which aims to develop new models for delivering care, will target patients whose needs have been neglected by traditional services. (Gulland, 1998a, p. 14)

Despite a crippling economic blockade, Cuba has reached World Health Organization targets ahead of London and New York. ...Health workers, not wanting to see their achievements destroyed, have proved ever resourceful, turning to 'green' medicine and acupuncture. Some Cuban health workers have become skilled at cannibalising redundant equipment to repair machinery needed to care for the patients. (Quick, 1997, p. 17)

Better outcomes and shorter hospital stays resulted when nurses were given greater autonomy or better skill mixes. (Kenny, 1997, p. 7)

Nurses have long understood the importance of health promotion but they have usually had to do it without organisational support. (Fielding and Woan, 1998, p. 36)

This miscellany of quotes points to the very diverse knowledge that nurses have accumulated and make available to individuals and society. As with so much else in nursing, this is frequently taken for granted by employers and politicians alike. Indeed, nurses themselves seem to be like squirrels, collecting information and knowledge and then storing it – perhaps often forgetting about it. In this way, we help neither ourselves, nor our clients and patients, nor indeed society at large. We are literally hiding our light under a bushel. This need not be so.

We should not forget that Florence Nightingale spent many years of her life collecting information and data on many subjects that proved essential to the construction of hospitals and the shape of health care in her day and long beyond it. With her team of nurses, she 'reduced the Crimean War hospital death rate from 42 per cent to 2 per cent (*The Wordsworth Dictionary of Biography*, 1994, p. 318). Nightingale had a very clear vision, and she kept to it, thus ensuring that she will be remembered for a long time yet. We may not like all the consequences of this vision today. As people with the same basic ideals, we are not called to be *imitators* of Nightingale but, like her, to be aware of the needs of the day and of the future.

Knowledge, being associated with mind, must be one of those concepts that Oppenheimer (1995) calls a 'bridge' between fact and value. We mind terribly about the knowledge we have; therefore it matters terribly to us. This knowledge, however, is not just a fact but is entirely bound up with the values of nursing. This is evident from the move into higher education. We now place more value on higher education, and the knowledge base has therefore taken a leap forward, becoming broader and also more specialised. We are concerned about this, worry about it, are proud of it and defend it. It matters to us; we mind about the knowledge we have. Our knowledge is our biggest asset and that which defines us as professionals. Having knowledge also makes us responsible in sharing it.

In the debate on professionalism, knowledge is a vital aspect. It matters *that* we have knowledge, *what* knowledge we have and *how* we use it. Communication is the major issue on which nursing as a profession depends. A profession is recognised by an 'extra dimension', which is that its members share with their clients what they have (Tschudin, 1992, p. 128). Perhaps what I am pointing to here is that nursing now needs to share its knowledge not only with its clients, but also with society at large. As long as politicians and policy makers have control over nursing, rather than nurses themselves, they need to be clear why nursing minds about its knowledge. The knowledge that nurses have can literally make all the difference. In small projects and in large islands like Cuba (referring to the quotes above), nurses make the difference.

That nurses have a great deal of knowledge is not disputed. Every person who comes into contact with a nurse prefers that nurse to have more rather than less knowledge. How that knowledge is used, however, matters. How nurses relate to the patients or clients who need care matters and will be remembered by them as much as will the actual technical skill. How the story of each person in such an

interaction is told matters. Even a simple act, such as
removing stitches, involves both people in the exchange
of important information.

Much nursing knowledge is empirical and therefore difficult to judge and value. This is part of the problem why disseminating nursing knowledge more generally is onerous. I would
argue, however, that for too long we have gone along with the
idea that knowledge must be able to be documented. Our
world is increasingly data based, to the exclusion of orally
transmitted knowledge. Yet, as human beings, we relate to
other human beings through our stories and our contacts more
than through our computer screens. We need to balance written
knowledge with that orally transmitted (Roberts, 1995, p. 216)
and often intuitive, psychological and spiritual knowledge that
is part of nursing as much as any other knowledge. The fact
that it is more difficult to document does not diminish this
type of knowledge; we must be clear about that.

Because this aspect of nursing is so strong yet also so difficult to access, it remains largely hidden. Nurses who have good
ideas cannot make them known because they sound, feel or
look impossible to someone concerned with evidence and
written plans. Intuition can only be taught by being recognised in others, yet intuition is over and over again the element
that saves patients' lives (Marks-Maran, 1997, pp. 92–108).
Perhaps in this area we should talk more about nursing 'wisdom'
rather than restricting everything to knowledge.

The hiding or concealing of knowledge can therefore
become a power game: if you don't want it openly, we use it
subversively. If you don't listen, we will not co-operate. Nursing
is full of incidents of power games, the most obvious one
being between nursing and medicine: two professions working
side by side yet seemingly constantly to be trying to outwit
each other. Heslop and Oates (1995, p. 257) argue that power
'is relational, that is, it operates in conditions of resistance'.
People are positively influenced and shaped by society and
by descriptions that are at the same time also restraining and
limiting. This may cause a shift in knowledge. Power and know-

ledge can then become productive and not only repressive. It is this possibility which may give nursing the leading edge in the future.

Sams (1998, p. 78) describes well how a trust's group of nurses concerned with palliative care used the 'bottom-up' method of distributing information. This was not only beneficial to the group concerned, but also finally made an impact at the Department of Health (DoH). Such stories are encouraging. They should, however, be not the exception but the rule.

Nursing knowledge has to be used for evidence, but it also has to be used professionally. If the hallmark of a profession is that it shares what it has with its clients, knowledge is clearly the most obvious element to share. When knowledge is 'liberated' from its use as power, it can become creative. It may be argued that this is altruism and might mean a loss of distinction in nursing. However, the experience of all nurses, and people generally, is that what is shared is not lost, rather, something more is gained by it. Sharing is not simply saying, 'I give you half of what I have', but involves us as human beings. We can only become 'more' human when our relationships are creative.

> The knowledge that nursing has is vital, and if nurses are to matter, they need to mind about the knowledge they have and dare much more to disseminate and share it. Only in this way will nurses themselves, nursing as a profession and society at large be healthier and 'better'.

Our professionalism matters

Cheek and Rudge (1995, p. 323) write about professionalism in nursing from a feminist perspective. They point to the fact that women are not so much concerned with 'the knowing subject and the known subject' as with 'consciousness raising'. They say that:

> The notion of 'raising' is a metaphor for the emergence of an awareness that, once it had surfaced, allowed the possibility for action

to occur. In nursing's case, one of the possible benefits of conscious-ness raising is to enable nurses to see the multiplicity of points at which they can resist the various forms and guises of power that are embedded in nurses' oppression.

The authors describe the known model of professionalism as 'patriarchal', which is 'based on the hegemony of the analytic discourse of the "expert" which is viewed as being derived from a legitimate knowledge base which is then used to legit-imise the power and practice of that professional group'. The inference is that, for women (and nursing, which largely comprises women), this model is not well suited. In nursing, with a large oral culture – stories of suffering, intuition and handover reports – the personal is devalued.

Davies (1996a, p. 46) also sees professionalism in terms of gender differences. She says that the classic way of being profes-sional – 'all-knowing, distant and detached' – is masculine. Masculinity, she says, is:

> calmly evaluating the options, being strictly in control of self and, indeed, of others. For if the world is populated by other mascu-line selves, each with their individual projects, then there is little room for shared enthusiasms or co-operative activity.

Davies is careful to point out that it is not so much indiv-idual men who hold to these views, but that much of what is happening is still 'culturally understood'. When looking at these issues, this must be kept in mind.

I am not convinced that professionalism and professional practice necessarily equate. It is possible to have very high levels of professional practice and competence, but this does not necessarily mean that the profession is thereby enhanced.

Denner (1995, p. 27) asks whether, by cannulating patients and taking blood samples at night in the absence of a resident casualty officer, she is becoming more like a doctor's hand-maid or technical functionary. She has the knowledge and skills not only to perform the tasks, but also to judge that the tasks need doing (a high level of professional competence), but by the sheer doing of it, she is not advancing her profession because she is being taken advantage of. Professionalism can be a two-edged sword.

Macara (1997, p. 199) says that 'professionalism is the demonstration in practice of the aptitudes, attributes and attitudes to which practitioners lay claim and which might reasonably be demanded of them by those entrusted to their care, and by their colleagues of good repute and competency'. In a response to Davies' (1996a, b) articles, Macara (1996, p. 46) does not like the argument on gender and points out that the medical profession is concerned with updating and developing the ancient virtues of medical professionalism. These have been formed into core values for all health professionals: 'commitment, caring, compassion, integrity, competence, spirit of inquiry, confidentiality, responsibility and advocacy'. It is striking to note that these values, which the medical profession is widely and proudly advocating, are essentially the same as those formulated for the nursing profession by Roach (1992) (see above) as long ago as 1984.

Guidelines, codes, regulations and ever more specific interpretations of them (UKCC, 1998a) aim to ensure that the public is protected through professional standards. In these days of the constant threat of legal action if a mistake is made, this is surely necessary. At the same time, it is also a belittling of the individual's intelligence and professional decision making.

In her paper on professionalism, Davies (1996b, p. 55) suggests that a 'new' professionalism is called for. She points in particular to the shift of emphasis that preceptorship, mentoring and clinical supervision create. These elements encourage individual responsibility and develop standards that are less rigid, seeing care as a team phenomenon, 'drawing out and enhancing the contribution of others, whatever their formal roles and titles'. Needless to say, this immediately questions 'how a collective can be held to account when the boundaries between professions and between professionals and non-professionals remain as strong as they are today'.

Given these points, what professionalism is clearly needs to be discussed and constantly reformulated. This is what is happening anyway, but I would argue here that all of us need to be involved in this process and that it should not be left to researchers, academics or the UKCC. As individuals, we have our personal and professional boundaries. Most people are only vaguely aware of where their boundaries are, and they therefore they never reach the real boundaries, stopping well short of them. When we do know our boundaries, we can go as far as the limits and push them out as and when necessary. Professionalism is also recognising our professional boundaries and then pushing at them. It matters that we care about professionalism and that we put it at the centre of nursing. However, we maybe need not simply go along with the accepted view of what it means. Part of this pushing at the boundaries is about looking forward and sideways, experimenting with new ideas and experiences, and sharing these with colleagues and clients. When we know our centre, we can spread to the limit and come back again. It is this which matters and which we mind about.

In 1994 the DoH issued its report *The Challenges for Nursing and Midwifery in the 21st Century,* listing there (p. 21) what the contributors call 'The nursing constant', that is, core skills and values that remain constant in nursing while the role of the nurse evolves. These constants are:

- a co-ordinating function
- a teaching function, for carers, patients and professionals
- developing and maintaining programmes of care
- technical expertise, exercised personally or through others
- concern for the ill, and also for those currently well
- a special responsibility for the frail and the vulnerable.

When we can hold on to these core values and develop them, then, I believe, the professionalism in and of nursing will have advanced. This is the business of every nurse.

'Mattering matters': it matters that what we care most deeply about is taken seriously and given full weight. It matters that we, as nurses, are aware of our treasures and our gifts, many of which cannot be weighed, measured or analysed into statistics, nor rewarded with money. When we mind about these things, we do indeed bridge a gap between facts and values because both of these aspects matter equally, albeit often in different proportions. When we are sure of their worth, we are more easily able to value them ourselves and make our values known to those who see differently from us and would therefore belittle or devalue what matters to us. It is no longer valid that the work – all the work – of nurses is treated as of less worth than that of other professionals in the health care field because it cannot be measured and compared with tools of scientific measurement. Nurses themselves are the tools in some areas. To help others to see this, we must be sure that we first believe it ourselves and trust ourselves enough to defend this stand. The idea that people matter can only be put into practice when we acknowledge that what matters to people matters.

4

Mattering is More Given than Chosen

In a society where we have light and power at the throw of a switch, instant coffee and access to any information world-wide, we find it difficult to deal with elements that are beyond our control yet are also the closest to us. When faced with these elements, our values become apparent, and our actions and reactions reveal our personality: who and what we are and where we come from. The following quotes give an inkling of what is involved:

> Where you live [in Britain] is more important in assessing your chances of dying in the early 1990s than it has been at any time since World War II. (Joseph Rowntree Foundation, 1997)

> There is nothing wrong with the country or the people; it is the government which is corrupt. (said about Pakistan on BBC Radio 4, *Today*, 14 August 1997)

> The meaning of our existence is not invented by ourselves, but rather detected. We can discover this meaning in life... by doing a deed, by experiencing a value, by suffering. (Frankl, 1962, pp. 101, 113)

If we want to assert that people matter and that what they are about – what they mind about – matters, it is also important that we understand *why* these things matter to people. What matters to us above all are the things we 'should' be able to control but largely cannot: the ways of dying, because the environment is against us; the government that we have elected and now find is corrupt; the relationships that go sour and destroy families. We mind about our life, health, family and relationships, but these things are bigger than ourselves and we must grapple with their power.

More given than chosen

As the last two chapters dealt more specifically with the 'mechanics' of mattering, so this chapter considers the deeper basis for the thesis. While Oppenheimer (1995) deals with the philosophical grounding of her ideas in the part of her paper entitled 'Real mattering' (pp. 67–76), I will again use her words and ideas to consider the situation in nursing as I understand it.

Vast arrays in our daily life are beyond our control. We cannot choose our parents (although anthroposophists might disagree with this). We cannot choose where and how we are born. We cannot choose our skin colour, our blood group, the weather, our neighbours and the *milieu* in which we are brought up. Indeed:

> Basic to human experience... is how little control we have over our life, the events that overtake us, the circumstances that surround us and even over that intimate part of us, our body. And what about our psychic, emotional life? How inexorably that reflects our inheritance, our conditioning. *We have been worked on before ever we were born, with no awareness, no consent of our own.* (Burrows, 1997, p. 98, emphasis added)

However, we also have much control over facts, because we clearly do influence our weather, our body and our emotional life. Choosing our skin colour, blood group and height and the sex of our children are near possibilities. We may have a choice over facts, but 'values are given to us' (Oppenheimer, 1995, p. 68). It is this fact that values are given to us which seems to be the problem, the challenge and indeed the purpose and meaning of much of what we are about.

Children cannot chose the circumstances in which they are brought up, and they are not capable of choosing the values by which they are surrounded. Both nature and nurture characterise us. Many – perhaps most – people then spend much energy throughout life in justifying, refuting or upholding the values that they recognise as their own and as worth defending and passing on to others. Frankl (1962) sees this as the search for meaning that is at the heart of our existence.

The elements over which we have no control are precisely those which form our character. The fact that we have to live with so many things that we cannot change means that we have to address these things in one way or another. Our morality is therefore addressed, as is our humanity in general. In order to be and remain human, we have to respond to people, objects and events.

We can choose our life partners, but we cannot choose how that partner's life develops. We can go on a journey, but we cannot choose how the driver or pilot of that journey will affect us. We can only respond to what is then given to us, and in this responding is revealed what matters to us. Oppenheimer (1995, p. 67) gives two examples of how mattering is perceived: 'My family has a claim upon me' and 'My wife brings out the best in me.' Both examples are recognisable for people, although quite what is being done and perceived is difficult or even impossible to describe. In a similar form, we could say within nursing that 'Our patients shape our character' or 'After working in that environment I am not the same person as before.' We recognise an influence on us as coming from other people and our environment, but how exactly this has come about is almost impossible to describe. We have not necessarily chosen that influence, but we have not hindered it either: we have at some level consented to it. If we asked 'my wife' or patient X how they thought they had influenced us, they might be astonished to think that they do or did in fact influence us.

If we have no choice over the beginnings of our lives, it is also true that, at the end of life, our choices diminish. Declining health, vigour and mental ability are largely outside our control, but the way in which we deal with them is not. An awareness of limitation, helplessness and dependence on others is very difficult to cope with for some people (although clearly not for others). Because these situations, people and events are 'given', they matter; for the time being, they are our 'mattering', and we 'mind' about them.

On a much wider scale, what are also 'given' in nursing are the culture, history, political and economic environment and scene. We have not chosen them, and we cannot undo what they have done. They have shaped our lives, and precisely because they are there, they matter to us. We have chosen nursing as a profession, and what concerns nursing – personally, professionally and socially – has to be our concern. The health care scene in which we work may be very different from the one we knew when we decided to start nursing. In our most personal caring, we are influenced by economics, and social policies dictate what we do or do not do in terms of treatment. Since they often oppose or contradict each other, we have to mind about them, deeply and constantly. When one value comes up against another, our real deepest sensitivities are challenged. In the response we make to such mattering lies our morality, our meaning and what our life is about.

Truth

Oppenheimer (1995, p. 73) calls truth, beauty and goodness the 'traditional ultimate values'. When applied to this book and this thesis, it becomes clear that they play a major part in our daily lives.

Oppenheimer distinguishes between 'moral truths' and 'factual truths'. She cites Walton (1994), who asks why there is science fiction but not morality fiction. Oppenheimer agrees with him that we cannot invent 'a morality like a time-travelling device' but also thinks that 'it would be a pity to underestimate our freedom to explore worlds which are not ours'. Oppenheimer (1995, p. 74) says that 'we can switch off our real factual beliefs and enter into a story about dragons and time travel more easily than we can accept a story about a miracle in a modern hospital'. What is it about miracles in modern hospitals that we cannot accept them as 'truth' when we have no problem accepting dragons as 'not truth'?

We accept many things as truth that we have no means of testing. In many instances, our means of testing are not applicable to certain 'facts'. We cannot measure psychological insights in the same way as we measure electricity, but we cannot deny the truth of the existence of both. Many people accept as truth anything that health professionals tell them. Stories abound of people still sticking to some diet 20 years after they were advised that eating or not eating something might be helpful. It is still difficult for many people to accept that there might be alternatives to care because they believe in the truth of the one possibility suggested. We now dismiss cures and treatments of earlier ages as myth and magic, but we are on the brink of discovering that our own scientific age may be far more unscientific than many of us would like to believe. Perhaps lifesaving equipment and medications are 'magic', in the sense not of working wonders for us but of being nothing more than an expensive piece of make believe (Wilkinson, 1998, p. 170).

Every nurse knows the devastation that the telling or otherwise of 'the truth' can cause. We are concerned with the fact of truth, which we understand to be the baseline for our functioning. It seems increasingly obvious, however, that our facts are not as adequate as we had imagined and that they are nowhere near enough. The moral truths of our lives are just as important, in many instances more so.

The moral truths – who we are and what we are – only become clear to us in the living of our lives. The individual stories (truths) fit into the wider picture of the prevailing story (truth) of the world around us, and it is in adjusting to these that we come face to face with moral truth.

The revealing and withholding of truth involves power. In nursing, this is often felt most keenly at times when nurses are not consulted, are brushed aside or overlooked as not being important, or are treated as servants. When nursing is downgraded, 'people (nurses) don't matter' seems to be the order of the day. For professionals who promote that 'people matter', to experience the opposite is perhaps one of the strongest reasons for the inability, which seems so pernicious, to have confidence in their own profession and value.

Perhaps the most obvious people who brush nurses aside in this way are doctors. Nurses and doctors work so closely with each other that the relationship they have needs to be constantly considered and renewed. However, I think that far more all-pervasive is the attitude of policy makers and politicians. Anyone in charge of large groups of people (including managers) is liable to use his or her power to disregard the needs of the people concerned. Decisions made without consultation mean that moral truths are not taken into consideration. This diminishes both sides of a relationship.

Truth is not some 'item' that can be added or left out according to circumstances. Like empathy or compassion, truth is not some thing but is 'a way of being'. It is not a question of telling or saying the truth, but of acting truthfully and living honestly. When people matter, this aspect becomes central. The language used here – of mattering and minding – can therefore be seen even more to bridge fact and value.

Trust is generally regarded as a consequence of truthfulness. When truth is told, trust follows. Faulder (1985, p. 26) asks:

> why is it that trust is almost uniquely discussed in terms of the patient's confidence in the doctor? Seldom do we hear about doctors trusting their patients by, for example, allowing them to see their medical records.

One can take this analogy further and ask why nurses (and people generally) should feel that they need to trust those in authority, but similarly those in authority do not trust those of whom they are in charge. With tongue in cheek, Pattison (1997, p. 129) advises managers on how to manage badly, saying (among other things):

> Be surprised and hurt when other groups and people attack or question your intentions and good faith. This helps people to create a communication barrier and may prevent awkward questions from the citizenry being asked or taken seriously.

Truth and trust are not one-way streets.

Truth can very easily become *the* truth, that is, a principle or an idea that must be believed and adhered to. Gilligan (1982, pp. 104-5) considers Gandhi, who, in the guise of love, imposed 'his truth on others without awareness of or regard for the extent to which he thereby did violence to their integrity'. She considers this to be sacrificing people to truth. However, she also states that both non-violence (which Gandhi practised) and psychoanalysis share a commitment to seeing life as an 'experiment in truth' (p. 104).

It perhaps therefore becomes possible to say that to affirm that 'people matter' is also an experiment in truth. When seen as an experiment – something that we consciously try – there is no longer the need to hold on to power of any kind, sharing becoming the *modus vivendi*. This takes courage, but it is essentially the only way to work ethically. Truth is then not just a fact but a process, and this is yet another way in which 'mattering matters' bridges fact and value.

The 'shadow' side of truth is that nurses have been reluctant to volunteer their 'truth': the truth that they matter and need to be considered as equal partners with their professional colleagues. The given facts of this situation are well known: the climate of nursing in general and the status of women in particular. However, the climate *is* now changing, and we can no longer simply sit back and bemoan the situation. If we want to remain a viable entity as a profession, we have to act as ethical beings. The situation is given: we have not chosen it (or may only have chosen it in so far as we have chosen nursing). In the words of this thesis, however, it matters to us, and it affects us. We mind about it, and therefore it matters. Our deepest values are addressed and questioned, and this leads us to act differently and to change the climate for those who come after us. This is ethical – good – acting.

Goodness and beauty

In considering goodness and beauty under the same heading, Oppenheimer (1995, pp. 74–6) uses the word 'creativity' as a link:

> I believe that the principle 'people matter', as well as being important in its own right, might with care suggest a first step towards fitting creativity into the same system as moral goodness.

Because people mind about themselves and others, they matter. The kind of minding they do can also be called loving. Oppenheimer (1995, p. 75) says that:

> love cannot exist in a vacuum but has to be made actual in some sort of specific activity. As soon as we give love something to do we open the way to other valid concerns besides being good.

Beauty is not only art such as paintings, music, theatre and buildings. Sidgwick (1907, p. 400) believed that beauty was a necessary part of conscious life, along with virtue, truth and freedom. Finnis (1980, p. 89), however, comes closer to Oppenheimer' view:

> Aesthetic experience... need not involve an action of one's own; what is sought after and valued for its own sake may simply be the beautiful form 'outside' one, and the 'inner' experience of appreciation of its beauty. But often enough the valued experience is found in the *creation* [emphasis added] and/or active appreciation of some *work* [original emphasis] of significant and satisfying form.

Castledine (1998, p. 493) says that 'the art of nursing is about applying imaginative skill to human interactive situations'. Castledine is using the word 'art' to stand for the skill of creating relationships as well as for the production of beauty. If holistic care is the aim of all nursing practice, we cannot restrict such practice simply to the actual care given but must indeed consider the whole person. Evans (1997, p. 22) gives an example of such care to a dying patient in a hospice:

> I have seen patients change physically. One was curled up in a ball facing the wall, taking no interest in anything. A nurse went to be with her for a few nights, not worried about rejection or silence. Others had tried and failed, but this nurse either said the right thing at the right time or was simply just there. The patient went on to shine, literally – she talked and chatted and her room began to sparkle with all the work from her new hobby of painting on glass.

Here one can say that beautiful objects – paintings on glass – were the indirect outcome of a relationship between the nurse and the patient that was creative. One can say that the nurse was creative in achieving this relationship. It is therefore possible to say that the nurse was moral because she acted creatively. However, I doubt if this nurse could foresee what might happen because she sat with this patient for a few nights. What is much more possible to say is that the nurse was not afraid, was not looking for something and was not concerned about possibly being rejected. It is possible to say what is *not* there rather than what is. This *via negativa* was well known to medieval writers, and in matters of morality it seems to have a place. We can be more aware of what is given and present experience rather than choose what we want. Thus beauty and goodness only come about because we can act creatively. When we are not afraid, we act creatively; when we listen to hear, we act creatively; when we 'love our neighbour', we act creatively: in this way, beauty and goodness become values that are basic to all our actions. The nurse above minded enough about this patient – loved the patient – and the patient literally became a work of art herself by 'shining', and becoming creative with her painting. In her creativeness, the nurse brought forth goodness. These two people confirm what Oppenheimer (1995, p. 76) says she is 'feeling after', namely 'the idea that at last "beauty" or "the aesthetic" or even "pleasure" can take its place as the substance of the good life. Then we might say that goodness is its form; and truth, that is reality, its condition.'

Attending

Most writers on philosophy in the West have discussed truth, beauty and goodness for one reason or another. Eastern philosophies have concentrated on the notions of identity of the individual self (*atman*) and the absolute (*Brahman*). This leads to the knowledge that there is only one reality. Be they Eastern or Western philosophies, or cultures from north or south, what they all have in common is their search for truth and for the acquisition of the values that lead us in the search. If what matters to us is valuable, can we be right or wrong about values? Can people be right or wrong about what matters to them? Oppenheimer (1995, p. 69) says yes, with a hint of apology in her voice. She says that:

> we find values by *attending*. If people find different values, we can allow for different points of view. We can compare moral disagreements with the well-known problems of perception, the straight stick that looks bent in water, the elliptical penny, the train moving away and getting smaller... Rose-coloured spectacles can be literal or metaphorical. Some of us see better than others, and anybody's vision can be distorted in various comprehensible ways. (original emphasis)

All of us see what we want to see and hear what we want to hear. However, if values are given to us rather than chosen, is it possible to say that we make distinctions between what we hold as valid and what we choose to be valid? With so many influences upon us every day, it is almost impossible to say that we choose something completely autonomously while other events or items influence us. Perhaps the word 'find' needs to be clarified in this context. We may indeed go looking for certain ideas, ideals and truths, and then we find something that fits our frame of reference. In this way, our 'finding' has been an active search. Probably more often, however, we happen to come across something and recognise it as 'true' or 'good' for us, this 'finding' being completely serendipitous. Clearly, the two paths overlap. If the whole of life is an 'experiment in truth', the values that we 'find' as we live are all part of this search.

An 'experiment' means that we attend to what is happening, and we can only recognise something as being of value if we have paid attention to it. It may therefore be possible to say that the experiment consists in attending, and when we attend to people, events and places, certain things can happen to us.

I have no doubt that, for most people, an illness or accident is such a time of attending. The inevitable question – why did this happen? – can be explained only to a certain extent by circumstances. Beyond a few facts, such as having crossed a road or taken a particular risk, we are in the realm of personal knowledge, values, meaning and truth *vis-à-vis* ourselves and others. We are faced with our own vulnerability and unpredictability and the shadows with which we would rather not have to deal. When caring holistically for patients and clients, we may therefore have to pay much more attention to what is happening to them in terms of insights, shifts in values, and the emotional powers to heal or the blocks to such healing. Elsewhere (Tschudin, 1995), I have written of the importance of questions in such situations. The two main questions that may indeed need to be asked are 'What is happening?' and 'What is the meaning of it?' It may need a more personal question, such as 'What is going on for you at this moment?' or 'Is there any sense or meaning for you in what is happening to you?' The questions may not need to be asked as such, because in many conversations, we touch on the meaning or core of the person anyway. The important thing is that we hear what is being said and reflect this empathically. This, surely, is attending on the part of the nurse, allowing the client or patient to attend also to him- or herself. When we pay attention to a person in need, we literally change the world.

An example of this is a personal experience. At a workshop some years ago in a church hall, I was outlining these questions. When I touched on the centrality of the question 'What is the meaning of it?', an elderly man shot up from his seat and said, 'If someone had asked me this question 30 years ago, my life would have been different.' I do not know what 'the problem' was nor what meaning this man suddenly made of it, but he had clearly 'found' some value for something that had eluded him all this time. I did not give him the meaning, and I did not even attend to him in particular; I can merely say that I was a kind of midwife – and the job of midwives is to 'attend' to people as they give birth. Maybe asking patients or clients what meaning an illness or disease has for them can be the key that unlocks the door to understanding and coping in new ways.

Another metaphor for the attention, which is so necessary in understanding this idea, is that of the carpenter, working a piece of wood with the grain. Working with the grain shapes and forms the object. Sooner or later, there will come a moment of meeting a knot, and it is then that a decision will have to be made on whether the knot is to be taken out or included, and how. Similarly, our lives are formed and shaped by so many influences of which we may be barely aware until we come to some point of difficulty. Only then do we realise who or what we are, and we need to face ourselves. When we are either able alone to pay the necessary attention or are helped to do so, we can see that what has gone before is valuable and necessary. What we may need now and in the future may reveal itself through the attention we now give. In the words of an anonymous saying:

> Raise the stone and you will find me; cleave the wood and I am there.

Perhaps this slight detour was necessary to highlight the important point that 'objective values look much more convincing when we posit, not *something that* matters, but *someone who*'. (Oppenheimer, 1995, p. 69, original emphasis). It is in paying attention to people (attending to people) that we really recognise what matters. Values are valid because they matter in relation to people rather than only as facts: things matter in relation to people.

> People matter, in the strongest sense of mattering; they matter in their own right; things matter in relation to people. (Oppenheimer, 1995, p. 69)

Oppenheimer goes on to say that 'this is where love comes in: the mattering of people cannot be separated off from the interconnectedness of their minding' (p. 69). Mattering is indeed more given than chosen, and with love we touch on what matters, and we influence the choices we make.

Shadow and archetypes

In order to understand some of the 'real mattering' in nursing, it will be helpful to consider here certain aspects of nurses and nursing from the point of view of the archetypes and the shadow as they have come to be described in psychology. C.G. Jung (1875–1961) made great use of them in his work. He described archetypes as 'archaic remnants', 'primordial images', 'collective images' (1964, p. 69) and 'collective representations' (1964, p. 42). Gordon (undated, p. 7) says that Jung linked archetypes:

> directly to instincts. He described them as psychosomatic entities, whose physical expression is instinctual action, reaction and behaviour, while their mental expression is in the form of images.

According to Stewart (1992, p. 252), the 'shadow involves the personal unconscious, instincts, the collective unconscious and archetypes'. They are made evident in 'both negative and positive projections, which are powerful and potentially destructive', but which a person can be helped to own, accept and integrate, thus breaking their compulsive hold.

The terms 'shadow' and 'archetype' are associated with strong negative or obscure connotations in popular understanding. They are sometimes used in association with each other and sometimes separately. I will concentrate more on the archetypes here. The negative indication of archetypes is largely a result of fear of their powers. Some of the values and mattering discussed above have deep roots in archetypes.

Archetypes are the essence of dreams, tales, stories and the personal unconscious. The archetype of the nurse represents both the woman and the mother who nourishes. As this is symbolic language, gender is not as differentiated as it is in practice. There is a possible confusion with a child's (wet) nurse and a sick nurse, but the nurse is essentially identified with the 'anima', that is, with the unconscious female part of the man's psyche. The anima connotes the mother, sister, wife, daughter, the 'wise' woman, witch, the 'angel in white' and female ancestry and progeny in general. The nurse nourishes, protects and strengthens physical growth (the wet nurse) and promotes emotional growth (the sick nurse). Thus, the nurse is a healer in the broadest sense of the word, restoring, binding wounds, soothing heated brows and 'making good'.

In the woman's psyche, the nurse is her whole being. When this is not well recognised or accepted, the shadow of the archetype becomes evident. In this case, the nurse is the healer with the hard edge, who discriminates, withholds and is 'cruel to be kind'. She denies autonomy to her patients by keeping them dependent in a 'baby' condition, calling them 'pet' and 'sweety' to reinforce the fact. However, this is symbolism, yet we, in fact, too often recognise these very traits both in ourselves and in others being carried out. In (women) nurses, the shadow of the nurse can become personified and used with sinister effect.

Johnson (1977, p. 62) quotes a Chinese proverb:

> A man stands on the mountaintop at dawn and holds forth his hands, palms up, to say the creative yes. A woman stands on the mountaintop at dawn and holds forth her hands, palms down, to say the creative no.

Johnson says that the nature of women is to be generous, to be able to discriminate, to do one thing and do it well. At crucial moments, they also have to say no creatively. When women say no constantly, they are acting out of their negative masculinity rather than the archetype.

The instinct to curb, to stay with the known, to be 'all over the place' and not concentrate on the one thing needful is very strong in nursing. This represents the shadow of the shadow, the unfocused femininity and the aspect of the psyche that has not yet learned to say the *creative* no. Much of the historic legacy of nursing can be traced back to this element. In particular, the isolationism of nursing, the unwillingness to co-operate with other health colleagues, the maternalism with which junior nursing colleagues are treated, and especially the unwillingness to stand together when a colleague is in difficulty are part of the hard edge of nursing that withholds nurture and healing just when it seems to be needed most.

As nurses, we cannot help but be taken into the culture of nursing, and these values become part of us whether we want them to or not. They are given to us even when they are not chosen by us.

It is for me a very common experience when talking to a class of students and pointing out the responsibility that we have to change this culture to be faced with nurses always making much the same points:

- We cannot change the culture on our own
- One nurse cannot achieve anything
- I have tried but got nowhere
- Nurses cannot stick together
- The climate is too dangerous; better to keep your head down.

The body language that normally goes with such statements reinforces the message: the students tend to cross their arms in front of them, speak in a whiny voice and fix me with a look of 'Well, show us what you can do then.' If I challenge them, they become hostile. I would probably do the same in their position. However, with this stance, we only perpetuate the very strong myth that women are not much use, and this is not in any way helpful.

A part of the psychological development of all persons is learning how to deal with who and what we are. This includes the subconscious aspects of much of what our lives are about. When asked why people want to be or have become nurses, many of them say that they want to help people. Many of these people will not (at least not to begin with) realise that such a desire may be driven by a need to be helped themselves. The subconscious drive to get what we need is very strong. However, this is usually a futile search. It explains, however, why, sooner or later, most nurses become very disillusioned with nursing and perhaps leave. They may not be able to voice the fact that they had been looking for care, healing and support for themselves. The fact that they had not found them makes them sure that nursing is not for them. We do indeed not want to help and nurture our own when analysed with this yardstick. As nurses, we really have to learn to become nurses to ourselves first. We need to learn how to care for ourselves and protect, strengthen and restore our own psyche.

This is similarly true of all psychological aspects. Mothers have to be mothers to themselves, before they can be mothers in the true sense. Doctors have to be doctors to themselves, and lawyers have to deal with their own inner lawlessness by being lawyers to themselves before they can be true lawyers. One can take this a good deal further: who hasn't used the services of a plumber who tells us that he or she never gets round to doing the plumbing at home? This may sound trivial, and the psychological aspect of our work is more important in this analogy than the practical, but the two are so closely wound up with each other that they cannot be separated.

When we nurses learn how to be nurses to ourselves, we can then move forward. When we learn how to be nurses to ourselves and to each other, we become a force to be reckoned with. As nurses, we are the archetypal women who care, restore, nourish and protect. Johnson (1977) talks of four tasks that women have to perform in order to grow psychologically. These are the abilities to 'sort, to discriminate, to order' (p. 46); to be brave (p. 49); 'to do one thing and do it well'; (p. 57); and to say no (p. 63). The last task is the most difficult and may only need to be done infrequently. These tasks refer to the psychological growth and development of women and should therefore not be taken to apply to some specific task. However, it is clearly possible to say that nursing as a profession also has to go through these stages of growth. As nurses, we have learned to do the three first tasks particularly well over the centuries. The last task, saying no, may now be asked of us in a much more dramatic fashion. We need to be courageous and stick to this one task in order to achieve our goal. Then, when nursing is threatened – as I believe it is at present – by political and economic interference, the collective 'no' will be spoken with a strength of character that is quite irrefutable. Such a 'no' is not simply a contrary voice but is the voice of longing for goodness, driven by vision and justice.

I am mixing fact and metaphor with this language, but I am also sure that nurses reading this will recognise what I am saying. Because we recognise ourselves in such language, we mind about what is happening to us personally and to nursing generally. We are affected by all this, so it matters to us. This language, these metaphors, represent the bridge between fact and values as they are the 'application' of the theory described above. This 'mattering' is given to us by the fact of being nurses. We cannot change this, but our responsibility is to be creative, and in doing so we act morally. As citizens and as nurses, we are committed to each other as people by creating relationships in which we can grow. In nursing, our clients and patients are 'given' to us, that is, we have not chosen them. They challenge and enable us to search for what this means for nursing, and the most basic response to it must be simply that 'people matter'.

5

Saying Yes and Saying No

Saying 'no' is not simply a Luddite reaction. Women in particular have been associated with saying 'yes' at many different levels in their lives. Women who say 'no' are stereotypically seen as hard, ruthless, ambitious and egoistic. At the end of the last chapter, I quoted Johnson (1977), who believes that the essential task for women is saying 'no' – creatively. It is this which is essential. Simply saying 'no' can be destructive, but a creative 'no' is always for growth, at least psychologically.

In this chapter, I want to use this language and apply it also in areas such as health care. The foregoing chapters have laid the foundation on which such an argument can be based. What I propose here can only be considered in the light of the principle that people matter and that what they care and mind about matters.

Saying no

> Future generations will look back on these closing years of the twentieth century and call it the time of the Great Turning. It is the epochal shift from an industrial growth society, dependent on accelerating consumption of resources, to a life-sustaining society. (Macy, 1998, pp. 28–9)

Macy, a scholar of Buddhism and general systems theory, writes from this perspective and in this language. She writes that the Great Turning is happening at three simultaneous levels:

1. The actions in defence of Earth, which 'include all the political, legislative and legal work required to slow down the destruction of Earth'
2. Creating sustainable alternatives to the structural causes of the global crisis, such as local marketing and consumer co-operatives

3. The values to sustain such nascent institutions, which must mirror what we want and think we are. We have to open our senses 'to the web of relationships, in which we have our being'.

The 'turning' that is taking place is not a 'return' to the 'good old days' but a fundamental re-evaluation of much of our thinking and experiencing. Much of what has been promoted in the 20th century as good and profitable is now being questioned. Individualism, compartmentalising and specialising have pushed society forward in a direction that we now see as dangerous. We cannot separate ourselves from all that surrounds us. The 'turning' is recognising that, at every level, we are connected at far deeper levels than we might at times realise.

Not only in the economy and the environment, but also in the field of health care, do we have to learn to say 'no'. The level of care that we have come to expect from the NHS 'is idealistic – if you can find disease or defect we will try and cure it or prevent it. *Such a belief has very expensive consequences*' (Wilson, 1993, original emphasis). We may need to say 'no' to the splits between purchasers and providers because they divide rather than care and, via their extra administration, 'steal' precious resources. More strongly still, we can say that, because we treat death as a failure rather than as a reality, we try every way to correct the failure and ignore the reality. Illich (1976, p. 179) put it very starkly when he said, 'in every society the dominant image of death determines the prevalent concept of health'. Our efforts to delay death deplete our efforts to maintain and foster health. The consequences of trying to avoid death are gradually ruining the economic health of nations in the affluent societies. It is here too that we have to learn again how to say 'no'. However, it is not simply a 'no' after which nothing more can be said. Nor is it a 'no, but...': it is a 'no, and...'. The 'and' is in the sharing. We need again to 'turn' to sharing.

Radford Ruether (1983, p. 236) traces death-based religions to the time of the hunters and warriors. While men killed both animals and other humans and were in constant danger of being killed themselves, the experience of women was birth and the basic concern to nurture ongoing life. This resulted in birth-based religions. While all such divisions and comparisons are too simplistic, it is clearly obvious that our legacy of a death-based religion is still very influential in our Western culture and therefore in our thinking. The emphasis on preventing death may have roots far deeper than our present scientific age.

The realisation that we are in a time of transition is not restricted to health care and ecology. Undoubtedly, every other generation also considered itself to be at a turning point. The only thing that is different today is that we have speeded up the process of transition to such an extent that we can see the differences in a very short space of time.

One of the points made again and again, and for various reasons, by many individuals and groups is that we have taken so much out of the earth in terms of natural resources that we cannot go on in the same way without major problems. Not only do we need to reduce the extraction of resources, but also we must put something back into the earth for it to be able to continue to live, and us with it.

Hoda (1995, p. 10) quotes E.F. Schumacher, famous for his book *Small is Beautiful*, as saying (from private notes) that:

> it is now widely accepted that there are limits to growth on the established pattern, so that, in all probability, the trends established over the last twenty-five years could not be continued even if everybody wished to do so. The requisite physical resources are simply not there, and living nature all around us, the ecosystem, could not stand the strain. ...In fact, the truth is now dawning that the world cannot afford the USA, let alone the USA plus Europe plus Japan plus other highly industrialised countries.

The problem is that we do not want to give up anything to which we have now become accustomed. Some years ago, a slogan exhorted people to 'live simply so that others can simply live'. In the present climate, this seems altogether too patronising by inferring that 'others' can exist on very little and that they do not need more, while all we need to do is give up a few extras that we do not need anyway. Saying 'no' is something much more radical.

A good deal of it is already happening. Grove-White (1995, p. 24) writes of:

hundreds of thousands, indeed possibly millions, of people [who] are voting with their feet in favour of all kinds of new perspectives, in favour of new complementary or alternative medicines and therapies, based on radically different and more modest assumptions about health, about the body, indeed about how the human person actually works in relationship with others – about death – radically different from the definitions embedded in conventional scientific medicine. It is startling how this dimension of cultural change has been so absent from... crucial political debates in recent years.

Worth (1997, p. 3), Director of Public Health in Huddersfield, Yorkshire, advocated the use of complementary therapies because of various contributory factors:

Firstly, the many therapies which command a range of attitudes with the health system from 'acceptable' to 'misunderstood'. Secondly, the declining public faith in the NHS and *conventional western medicine*. Thirdly, our increasing expectations of longevity and comfort which conventional health systems are unable to meet and finally, the role of highly placed 'champions' assigned to complementary therapies as a whole, e.g. HRH The Prince of Wales. (emphasis added)

An aspect of this move has no doubt to do with the fact that medicine as it was known and practised in the mid-20th century was centred on hospitals and institutions, enabling a strong control of practice, requiring compliance and concentrating largely on pathology. This is clearly no longer acceptable. The quotations above are ample proof that people today are looking for a different kind of care that takes into account the whole person and enhances the person rather than attacking a disease. The awareness has been growing steadily that, as humans, we are not so much the masters of our world as the stewards of it; this includes the view that we can only use our rights to the degree that we are responsible. Indeed, the Prince of Wales has been quoted as saying that:

we live in an age of rights. It seems to me that it is about time our Creator had rights too. I believe we have now reached a moral and ethical watershed beyond which we venture into realms that belong to God. (Linzey, 1997, p. 21)

It is the growing awareness that medicine has to be 'responsible' in the sense that it is not only successful, but also appropriate to the individuals it treats. Roszak (1995, p. 251) speaks of:

scrutinizing the trees and ignoring the forest, ...scrutinizing the cells and ignoring the organism, ...scrutinizing the detailed minutiae of experience and ignoring the whole that gives the constituent parts their greater meaning.

It is this, he says, which has made us 'ever more learnedly stupid'. However, it is also this which is now making us clever again.

Cassell (1993, p. 32) makes similar points. He says that:

Technology is not the problem; it is the relationship to it of those who employ it that is problematic. If this is not solvable, our entire project is a waste of time.

He is clear that 'technology runs doctors rather than vice versa' (p. 36). The technologies (Cassell mentions 'PET scanners, MRI, angioplasty, endoscopy, automated chemistry machines, and so on – the whole wondrous parade'; p. 33) cause physicians to 'wonder' and be enthralled by the lure of the immediate and the unambiguous information. The real culprits, Cassell (p. 39) says, however, 'are the doctors who use it, the public who love it, and the narrow knowledge on which it is based'. He concludes that to this end:

we must learn how to teach doctors, who are in themselves the primary instruments of diagnosis and treatment, to tolerate uncertainty, accept ambiguity, deal with the complex, and turn away from mere wonder. (p. 39)

This in itself is a 'task for decades'.

Much of what these various texts point to is a need to say 'no'. I mean here as much a moral and personal 'no' as an economic one. Simply because we have the machines does not mean that we have to use them for everybody. Simply because a treatment is possible does not mean that I have to have it. Simply because it is there does not mean that it is good.

In recent years, we have come to hear a great deal about rationing and about people being denied the right to have a certain treatment because it would be too costly. When new drugs are available for certain conditions, such as multiple sclerosis, we hear of one person on this side of the street being able to have it because her health authority will pay for it and another person living on the other side of the street not able to have it because he lives in another health authority. This is clearly not just, and people are rightly indignant about it. However, if both people were in the position of having all the information available to them and having as much detail explained as any health professional knew, they could make the decision for themselves of whether or not they needed the drug. In this way, they would feel empowered and responsible rather than feeling disempowered by a system that, on the face of it, makes decisions on an arbitrary basis.

There will always have to be checks and balances in health care, but the various systems in existence, such as QALYs (quality-assured life years), total quality control and quality circles, are tools of management that seem a good idea when applied, except when they are applied to me. When it comes to the individual person, what matters is that the person is in control rather than a policy, however feasible it sounds or however 'nice' the person is who carries it out.

There are obviously plenty of situations in which individuals are not able to be in control or do not want to be, for whatever reason. This is too complicated and lengthy a topic to be addressed here. However, increasing situations come to light in which individuals have not been given the opportunity to be in control. Stories abound of mothers asking that a child should not be put through more trauma, of women having caesarean sections against their will, of dying patients being given chemotherapy without wanting it, of people being resuscitated when families have requested that they should not be. Yes, the climate is changing, but still the patients and clients are not heard enough at the level of 'people matter' and that what matters to them, matters.

Some form of rationing is not only reasonable, but also desirable. The experiment in Oregon, USA (Campbell, 1993, pp. 6–7; Talento, 1995, p. 144) has, however, not proved to be the 'cure-all' initially thought possible. Rationing is not simply a matter of economics but has to consider far more widely the aspects of personal responsibility and common morality. A small but important example of this is the directive from the NHS Centre for Reviews and Dissemination concerning cholesterol-lowering drugs. These drugs should only be offered as a last resort, and patients 'should first be encouraged to stop smoking, take exercise and improve their diet' (McTaggart, 1998, p. 9). The mismatch between expectations ('a pill for every ill') and personal responsibility for health is wide. Callahan (1994, p. 28) puts this in terms of ethics by pointing out that bioethics:

> has failed to pursue with sufficient imagination the idea of the common good, or public interest, on the one hand, and that of personal responsibility, or the moral uses of individual choice, on the other. By its tendency to reduce the problem of the common good to justice, and the individual moral life to the gaining of autonomy, it has left a moral void.

Our tendency to separate our life into different boxes means that we are now often in situations where, as individuals and as communities and nations, we are powerless to make a point or influence people as people and societies.

One of the main reasons for the attraction of complementary and alternative therapies is that people are in control in choosing the practitioner and the therapy. The increased time given to clients also means that there is much more interaction between client and practitioner. On the whole, such practitioners are not members of large institutions and do not have to defend a system. All this makes it possible for clients to be much more personally involved and in control, to be able to be responsible personally and, by choosing this path, to be voting with their feet and thus forcing a change of views and direction, hopefully for the common good.

The argument that making use of complementary and alternative therapies pushes individualism and personal autonomy to the extreme is only partially correct. These therapies generally involve people in an awareness of their surroundings, relationships and total way of living far more than does conventional medicine. When people engage with these different views and ideals, their relationship with themselves changes, thus addressing the personal and cultural need, and longing for change and for their own need to say 'no'.

Saying yes

If we should say 'no' to too much or too little treatment, we clearly need to say 'yes' to anything that is giving quality of life. The immediate dilemma for all health carers is often in deciding when life is no longer – or will never be – of quality.

People who turn to different forms of treatment have, in that very act, said 'yes' to a new way of thinking, acting and valuing. They have taken an active step, perhaps outside the known and safe medical environment. They may also have committed themselves financially in a radical way. They will have experienced the satisfaction of an engagement with their own health and well-being and perhaps that of their family. Yet, for the vast majority of people, such a step is simply not possible for the very financial reasons that give some people satisfaction. If we want any justice in health care, we need to learn above all how to involve the individual in decision making. This means much more exchange of information, listening to each other and respecting what we hear.

Wilson (1976, p. 70) writes of a little dialogue between a Buddhist monk and his master:

'What is the one ultimate word of truth?'
'Yes.'
'I asked, what is the one ultimate word of truth?'
'I am not deaf!'

Saying 'yes' in health care means assenting not only to treatments and care, but clearly also to the many issues surrounding this care. It means saying 'yes' to:

- the basic concept that people matter
- that what matters to people, matters
- the fact that what people mind about matters
- that listening is important
- that all concerned have their story to tell
- that each story needs to be heard and the person respected
- that the principle that people matter is accepted throughout an organisation or institution
- that this may involve change

- that the training of personnel may need to be revolutionised, with citizens ('ordinary' people) involved in curriculum design and content
- that there is a 'grass-roots' interchange between consumers and deliverers of care at a democratic rather than a hierarchical level
- that individual care and treatments should be far more negotiated (in every branch of care) rather than 'given', thus reducing problems of compliance, waste, frustration and disillusionment
- that issues of autonomy, justice, responsibility and the common good need to be discussed and balanced
- that the present as well as the future needs to be respected and imagined.

According to the International Council of Nurses' *Code for Nurses* (1972), the 'fundamental responsibility of the nurse is fourfold: to promote health, to prevent illness, to restore health and to alleviate suffering'. This can only be achieved with the co-operation of the individuals and communities concerned. It therefore requires consent – verbal or written, psychologically and morally. Yet how many times do we say 'yes' when we mean 'no'? We can be so easily manipulated into saying 'yes' and then regretting it but having no means of going back. How many of us have consented to some investigation, treatment or operation and, even while signing the consent form, felt uneasy about it? If we want to have the patient's or client's co-operation, we need to be sure that it is a wholehearted consent.

The point I am making here is that saying 'yes' in health care has to be for a quality of life that is recognised and accepted by all parties involved. If any party is not at ease with the fitting answer given or outcome sought in particular as well as general situations, then the answer cannot be 'yes'. We need to consider 'consent' in a much wider sense than is often the case at present.

When we are able to say 'no' to unnecessary or unethical treatments and care, especially concerning issues at the end of life, then we also have to be able (and enabled) to say 'yes' to death: our own death and that of others. (In end of life issues,

I also include decisions regarding very premature infants and those born at term with either congenital abnormality or an uncertain future.) Death is not simply a part of life but the most certain part of it. Wilson (1976, pp. 70–1) puts this in a thought-provoking way:

> The 'yes' to life and the future includes the 'yes' to biological death which comes to us from the hand of God as his given method of renewal and evolution. Each man [sic] dies that Man may grow towards his evolutionary fulfilment. My individual biological death demands of me the complete gift of myself, all that I am and all that I have, to the future of the whole creation. ...This means that my affirmation of another man – any other man – as my brother and not my rival demands of me (for completeness) a willingness to die that he may live.

This statement may sound old-fashioned and too altruistic for comfort. What we are seeing, however, is the practical application of this. When people are denied care because it costs too much, they may go to a national newspaper and make headline news, thus getting what they want, possibly depriving someone else of needed care. A person I was seeing for counselling some years ago, whose daughter was told that she needed a heart transplant, told me, 'Well, it's the Bank holiday, I hope that there will be lots of crashes that my daughter will get what she needs.' She will not have been the only person thinking like that. Our brother and sister may be very close to us. Put in these terms, an emphasis of 'I and Thou' is present, whereas my client saw more of an 'It' in a heart for her daughter. Perhaps, with Callahan (1994, p. 28), we need to 'work by looking both at individual responsibility and at the social dimension of the moral life' and then concepts such as 'brother' and 'sister' and 'I and Thou' take on a different dimension. Perhaps then the 'yes' becomes truly creative. Or, as Taylor (1972, p. 79) puts it, 'Truly to face death is to accept non-fulfilment and non-omnipotence as the very data of existence'.

Sharing

When people matter, we are sharing at a fundamental level by affirming that everybody matters: clients, nurses, doctors,

managers and politicians. Everyone matters equally. Each has
to tell her or his story, and each one's story has to be heard.
The stories have to be put together and compared and
contrasted. No one should 'win', and no one should 'lose', but
in each situation what is most fitting should be sought. For
patients, this may be 'no' far more often than hitherto seen.
For managers, it may be 'yes' to a decision that may need
more ingenuity and listening to their own workforce and attitudes than they have considered so far. Above all, for nurses,
it may have to be a willingness to share their knowledge with
their professional peers and relinquish the security that confor-
mity and hierarchy so often provide.

By sharing, I mean a fundamental sense of giving and taking
in equal measure. It seems that, so often, when health professionals reach the point in their training or education where
they know more than their clients, they lose the capacity to
share. They become conscious of power and use their power
to distance themselves. The following, which happened in 1997,
was related to me by a friend:

> L. had been in hospital for investigations and treatment of an
> intestinal complaint. One day a nurse brought her a tablet. When
> L. enquired what it was for, the nurse did not know and went to
> ask a staff nurse. She came back with the answer that it was a
> healing tablet. When L. enquired what it was called, she was reluc-
> tantly told the name. L. recognised that it was the brand name of
> a medication she had earlier taken and which had made her very
> ill. When she pointed this out, L. was told that the consultant had
> ordered it. The consultant had not discussed this with L. This
> episode made her feel betrayed and she was shattered at being let
> down by the consultant, whom she had hitherto respected and
> trusted, for not discussing her treatment with her, and the nurses
> for treating her in a manner which demeaned her personally and
> intellectually.

Unfortunately, such episodes will remain in patients' memories much more strongly than others that have been entirely
helpful and perhaps even the epitome of good care. A lack
of sharing – being with a human being as another human
being – is so often the only thing that is needed. Misunderstandings, small mistakes and a lack of attention happen to
all of us, but when we become aware of them and apologise

and are apologised to, most people are satisfied. In such inter-
changes, real humanity grows. However, when we feel the
need to justify ourselves, or to dismiss the other in order to
stay 'professional', we diminish ourselves and others. Such
situations are the ground – and rightly so – for complaints.
This leads to accusation and further justification, often leaving
neither side satisfied. Had we shared our humanity, we would
not only have avoided pain and hurt, but would also have
advanced human growth and friendship or perhaps even
gained a 'brother' or 'sister'.

When considering sharing, I do not mean a 'lady bountiful'
attitude. Giving to others out of our surplus is very laudable,
but it may not touch or affect us in any way. We share not
only our goods, but, just as importantly, also our time, thoughts,
feelings, knowledge and, above all, humanity.

Most of us also know from experience that those who are
rich give grudgingly and little; those who are poor share with
each other what they have. The sense of solidarity is the all-
important drive. What applies culturally can also apply personally and professionally. Nurses have always shared with their
patients and clients, both communities considering themselves
to be disadvantaged and 'poor'. When nurses can share generously with the 'rich' also, a new paradigm may appear because
they will be challenged in their attitudes.

When we as nurses share with our clients, it is this sense
of solidarity that drives us. Reams have been written about
how this happens and is possible. Noddings (1984, p. 34) says
that we:

> enter a feeling mode, but it is not necessarily an emotional mode.
> In such a mode we receive what-is-there as nearly as possible
> without evaluation or assessment. ...The one so engrossed is
> listening, looking, feeling.

Nortvedt (1998, p. 390) speaks of clinical observation with
an added dimension:

> Emotional receptivity reflects the nurse's experience of a patient's
> or his or her relatives' grief as an existing moral reality by which
> to be motivated.

Such moral responsibility is formed by the mere fact of being addressed by human experience.

What I mean by sharing, then, is an exchange, something given and taken not for gain or aggrandisement but from a sense of need because the other's need addresses me personally.

What do we share? I am concerned here with health care in particular, but since this touches all of life, I see vast areas where sharing needs to be much more of a reality. We need to share at the personal, organisational, local, national and international levels. At all these levels, we can do this only by 'listening, looking, feeling'. For this to be done, we need to tell our stories and we need to hear them. Yes, nurses need to listen to stories told by their clients, but, above all, nurses need to tell their stories in such a way that they *can be* heard and *are* heard. Many nurses tell their stories in research papers and articles, but how many of their managers read these papers and discuss them with the authors? How many nurses do not write anything all their lives and are never encouraged to be creative? Why are these nurses' stories never told and never heard?

We need to share at the local level. Galbally (1996, p. 342) says that 'training for health work needs to emphasize community and organizational approaches. Capacity-building should focus on the changing needs of specific environments and communities'. To do that, the focus must be 'on the social, cultural, political, legal, ethical and spiritual environments in which people live' (p. 341). How can we do this without listening to each other and respecting each other? People matter.

One important way of listening to each other takes place in 'schools'. Students of every kind, including those of nursing and medicine, are regularly addressed by patients and experts in various fields. This usually occurs in a 1-hour slot every now and again, after which the person goes home and the students may muse that it was 'interesting'. 'Patients' are not necessarily the best people to speak because they have a specific agenda. 'Citizens', on the other hand – 'ordinary' women and

men who may be the recipients of health care some day –
should be helping all students in health care to understand
local needs and priorities, exchanging with students at a daily
level so that the 'them' and 'us' divisions between givers and
receivers, experts and lay people, can never truly develop.
This is necessary not only in nursing and medical schools, but
also in training and learning institutions of every kind.

An important aspect of the peace process in Northern Ireland
was the need for all parties to listen to each other's stories in
detail and to hear what the 'truth' of the story was. Until this
was possible, each side told the world what the other's 'truth'
was as *they* saw it, not as the side concerned saw it. This meant
that the 'real' truth could never be heard. In each conflict,
there is a party that feels it is not taken seriously – just as
nurses feel that they are not taken seriously. In conflict, the
warring parties are 'siblings'. Conflicts only arise when close
brothers and sisters try to lay claim to the same inheritance.
'Cousins' do not fight, and they feel less involved with each
other. Nurses clearly feel themselves to be the 'wronged' sister,
not getting the same share of the attention and goods as their
'brother' doctors. Doctors cannot see what the fuss is about
because they do not similarly feel wronged. However, when
nursing makes advances and claims that might threaten medicine, the boot is on the other foot, and so the sibling rivalry
is perpetuated. We share an essential basic nature, and we
need to acknowledge this and dare to stop the vicious circle
by listening.

We need to share at the national and international level. All
of us become more aware of the global village with every picture
in the media of some other country's disaster. In order to be
effective internationally, we need to be active nationally. The
World Health Organization (WHO) has been very active in
the closing years of this century to make the 'Health for all
by 2000' strategy as valid as possible. Perhaps too late in the
day did it dawn on the strategists and politicians that the
century was rapidly running out and less had been achieved
than had been hoped. Oulton (1996, p. 344), the Chief Executive Officer of the ICN, wrote that 'complementarity must
receive renewed emphasis, and flexibility and tolerance must
become second nature to all health workers'. She does not

spell out what she means by complementarity, but one can hope that it means in large part a sharing between professionals at the deepest possible level.

The willingness to share is not simply another word for generosity or altruism. On the contrary, sharing is such a basic principle of survival that it becomes more and more the only possible way to live. The values that the market economy has given us have distorted our world view to such an extent that much of the Western world sees itself only in relation to itself. Some of the Western world's market 'gurus' have made famous U-turns, among them George Soros, the currency speculator and philanthropist. Having made his fortune on the back of a world-wide market crash, he has apparently argued that 'worship of the market place is undermining social values of morality and responsibility' (Positive News, 1997, p. 3). The world listens to him when he talks finance; will the world listen to him also when he talks morality?

Throughout the past few decades, various voices have made themselves heard fundamentally questioning the given order. Skolimowski (1994) describes as a set of cycles the various experiences that provided the Western mind with meaning. He recognises first Mythos, the Greek system of making sense of the world by the presence of gods. Out of this cycle grew Theos, the medieval world view that worshipped a transcendent divinity, leaving us its heritage of cathedrals pointing to heaven. With Bacon, Galileo, Descartes and Newton came the age of Mechanos. We are still governed by the ethos and culture of this world view while being aware that it is no longer sufficient. Reason (1998, p. 42–4) says that participation 'must be central to the new world-view' (p. 43). He uses the prefix 'co' to make some of his points: 'mind and the given cosmos are engaged in a co-creative dance' (p. 44); we all are engaged together in democratic dialogue as co-researchers and as co-subjects. In co-operative inquiry people work together' (p. 44). This is much the same point as Macy (1998, see above) made in her declaration that we are a 'turning'. If we do not learn to work together, we work against each other, and that is more quickly and globally destructive than any disaster. The many attempts to resolve conflicts that have been ongoing, often for years, is an encouraging sign. What is significant in such processes is that the parties together need to resolve their differences, usually with the help of a third party but not dictated by it.

How we share – as distinct from *what* we share – depends crucially on the situation and the parties involved. The first step is clearly a willingness to share and to reach a goal. An important aspect of any sharing (and conflict resolution) is that it is a process rather than a state. The commitment of all involved to such a process is vital.

> How we listen to each other matters. At this level, I believe, all the virtues known down the ages come into play. Listening takes patience, humility, a willingness to admit that one might have been wrong and make amends, gentleness, compassion, empathy, a non-judgemental attitude and believing the other person – to mention but a few. In other words, listening is a fundamentally ethical act. Sharing, therefore, can be said to be nothing less than a basic human activity.

Sharing in nursing

In a challenging situation, men tend to look for solutions and women tend to ask for more information (Noddings, 1984, p. 2). As sharing is so much about 'more information', it seems paradoxical that nursing, comprising so many women, has not made more of an impact in the arena of the world's health care. Sharing may therefore prove to be the challenge to nursing at this moment.

Sharing as a concept has long been used in industry in the idea of 'shared vision':

> IBM had 'service'; Polaroid had instant photography; Ford had public transportation for the masses and Apple had computing power for the masses. Although radically different in content and kind, all these organisations managed to bind people together around a common identity and a sense of destiny. (Senge, 1990, p. 9)

Senge (1990) describes at some length the need to see each other as colleagues in a team as this creates friendships. He says that (p. 245):

> as dialogue develops, team members will find this feeling of friend-ship developing even towards others with whom they do not have much in common. What is necessary... is the *willingness* to consider each other as colleagues. In addition, there is a certain vulnera-bility to holding assumptions in suspension. Treating each other as colleagues acknowledges the mutual risk and establishes a sense of safety in facing risk.

The need for sharing in nursing is certainly not new. The nursing process and nursing models have been early attempts to share care between nurses and patients. 'Collaborative working relationships' were words written into many Project 2000 programmes, and Rolfe (1996, p. 215) mentions 'collaborative inquiry' as an important part of the student-centred approach to learning and evaluating learning. Carlisle (1994, p. 15) des-cribes an organisation that started in the USA in 1978 'devoted to humanising institutions by putting the consumer at the centre of care', thus facilitating primary and team nursing.

The idea of shared governance has also been around for a while (Farrington and Geoghegan, 1995, pp. 734–5). These authors describe the philosophy of shared governance as empowering and partnering nurses to confront issues affecting their care in a better and more realistic way. This creates a framework for partnerships with other decision makers in the health care organisation. Gulland and Payne (1997, pp. 14–15) also see shared governance as a tool that can help to change the culture of nursing. They describe the pilot scheme at Leicester General Hospital NHS Trust, which adopted a 'council model':

> There are four different councils, each comprising up to 12 nurses, which concentrate on different areas – clinical practice, professional development, quality improvement and research. ...If a nurse has an idea about improving patient care or thinks something is not working she can approach a council member or fill in a sugges-tion form. The councils meet once a month and members take two hours out of work time to sit in meetings. Council chairs are allowed to take 10 hours a month, as they have to meet with fellow chairs.

In this model, nurses take turns by sitting on the council for one year only, thus potentially giving everyone a chance to appear in a decision making capacity.

Gulland and Payne do not say whether these councils only concern nurses or whether indeed the system is hospital-wide and includes all the various health professions. This would be the ideal situation. On the other hand, such councils would be very big and might possibly defeat the purpose again. This simply makes a further plea for the concept that 'small is beautiful', that is, that institutions and organisations need to be 'person friendly' and of such a size that the individual is never lost sight of. In such an atmosphere, individuals are able to engage with their work and take responsibility for further developments. From shared governance has come the idea of clinical governance (Chambers, 1998), and many other different ways of effective caring that may not yet be envisaged will surely follow.

What happens at the local level also needs to happen at the national and international levels. Nurses are often reluctant to become 'political', but what is political becomes personal with practice whether this is wanted or not. When we are sharing, we are less likely to make distinctions between spheres of work and thought, seeing wholes more than parts. 'Holistic' care also involves the work done at national and international levels. Reason (1998, p. 44) says that an important aspect of a participatory world-view is that it is about healing the alienation that characterises so much of modern experience. The disembodied qualities of modern life can be brought together again into a whole when we are able to share.

The possibilities for sharing in nursing and sharing nursing with others are limitless. Perhaps one of the most important places in which co-operation and collaboration are absolutely vital is in the education and training of health care personnel. All the various professions should receive as much as possible of their education together, not only in foundation courses and programmes, but also right throughout their professional education. Many of the specialised subjects, in particular the scientific subjects, are common to all professions. Far more important, however, are the subjects that cover communication and aspects of sociology and environmental and preven-

tive care. Most aspects of ethics and the law are also applicable to all students. Moreover, these subjects concern vital
aspects of decision making, either in terms of general rationing
or in individual cases, and the more the various professions
learn from the outset how to talk, discuss, consult and share,
the more patients and clients will eventually benefit. Some
attempts have clearly been made in terms of joint learning
and education, but, on the whole, vast areas still need to be
tackled, and the sooner the better.

Sharing enables people to be much more aware of their
possibilities and their limits. Sharing also enables people to
sharpen their moral acuity and become socially aware and
competent. In addition, sharing enables people to take responsibility and accountability more seriously. When we share –
because we *can* share – we become able to say 'no' and 'yes'
creatively. When we have reached the stage of authentic sharing,
we will have reached the possibility of genuinely and morally
saying 'no'.

Saying 'no' in nursing

As a group, nurses tend to say 'no' regularly when patients
are dying and the treatments ordered seem to make them
more ill rather than better. At this level, the 'no' is often a
clash of professional wits. Doctors are maintaining the
'preserving life' stance, and nurses are pointing to the fact that
they have more contact with patients and are thus in a better
position to judge what is needed. The clash is not over a moral
or ethical problem or dilemma but over who holds and main-
tains the moral high ground: the nurses or the doctors?

There will always be differences and clashes between personalities and individuals that will make such situations difficult.
It is, however, obvious that when the different professions
'grow up' together, they will see each other far more as
colleagues and friends rather than as an opposition or even
the immovable object that had to be countered with the irre-
sistible force. While the 'no' that nurses say in such situations
is now very often spoken in a defiant way, it becomes creative
when 'no' means 'I will not play this game any more; I will

treat my colleagues as friends; I will prepare the ground for dialogue and sharing; I will help my colleagues (nurses and doctors) to be creative too.'

There is no doubt that much of this is happening here and there, and this must be celebrated. As usual, such examples feel good and do good, and one wishes that they could be universal. When experienced nurses tell me that they are made to feel 'privileged' when they are consulted in decision making in intensive care units, it is clear, however, that it remains a wish. It is for this reason that nurses must tell their story loudly and clearly, and not be put off by feelings of unworthiness and modesty.

Part of the 'no' coming from nurses is also a sense of realism that much of the treatment and care of other than dying patients and clients is inappropriate. When nurses hear the stories told by clients, they hear tales of wrong diagnoses because they were not taken seriously, and often of much suffering inflicted for no clear purpose. Blood transfusions were given when simpler therapies were more indicated, and operations were carried out that were later discovered to have been unnecessary. Patients were given unrealistic hopes of organ transplants or pressured into accepting some care that they did not like or want.

The role of nurses is frequently that of 'translator' (Leners and Beardslee, 1997; Morrissey, 1997) from doctor to patient: explaining (and re-explaining) the diagnosis, prognosis and care, and informing doctors of what patients say, think and feel. This 'go-between' role is of crucial importance. It is often the third person that enables two parties to hear each other in disputes. In counselling, it is the third dimension – the relationship created between them – which is of importance to the two people involved. It is that 'spiritual' power which often opens our eyes or makes us aware of something 'more' that is happening. The role of the translator therefore needs to be taken very seriously.

I am firmly of the conviction that, when clients and patients are given far more information of the kind, and in the words and concepts, that they can understand, they can take into consideration their whole life rather than merely the disease. When this happens, they will say 'no' far more often and more readily to many 'treatments' and 'cures', and will want to live more whole and integrated rather than medically perfect lives. When they are helped to make such decisions, perhaps with the help of such a 'translator', they will return to dignity and autonomy far more readily than is now often the case. People who become dependent on a system from which there is no escape cannot be called free agents. Too many patients, however, feel trapped and unable to say 'no' and 'stop'.

On the other hand, plenty of elderly and incapacitated people feel an inner pressure to say 'no' so that they will no longer be a burden to families and society. It is a phenomenon of our age that those who cannot be productive cannot live. We make the equation 'productive = good', therefore 'unproductive = bad'. Such duality only leads us into corners of inhumanity, with too many people feeling useless and superfluous. All over the industrialised world, people are living longer, and we have to find the means of learning to live with our successes in such ways that they truly benefit us.

Patients must not be persuaded that 'no' is better than 'yes' or that they should say 'no'. Bringing aspects of economics and finance into any debate about decisions on health cannot be avoided, but if this is the only aspect, decisions have nothing to do with people, ethics, morality or responsibility. However, in order to be human and express our humanity, we need to decide on the basis of morality first and finance only a late second.

It is in situations of such decision making that nurses play a vital role. In listening to clients (patients, families, friends and colleagues), nurses hear what is being said. Perhaps more importantly, we hear what is *not* being said and is perhaps longing to be said. We may hear what hitherto might have been unspeakable. All this contributes to the story. Above all, it contributes to 'making' the person. New awareness and insights may be helping a person to experience for the first time what she or he has been trying to be. The person who is thankful for a cancer or suddenly 'finds' him- or herself after a heart attack may now need to take some drastic decisions, and they may have little to do with the kind of care or cure offered, despite needing to take it into consideration. Such people may need much support, and it is here that the need for the creative 'no' for women and the feminine aspects of the personality come into play most clearly. The advocacy roles that many nurses now feel to be theirs may be just what is needed. However, I would also urge caution, as the role can easily be misused, nurses projecting on to their clients their own inner needs to say 'no' and thus inadvertently being unhelpful or even destructive. It is for this reason that I have stressed self-awareness as a necessary element in all caring, and knowledge of the archetype and shadow of the nurse as being vitally important.

When nurses help clients and patients to say 'no' – and they may have to do this increasingly – they are involved in a job that is clearly bigger than the immediately obvious. In such situations, the two people concerned are in the process of enlarging the human sphere of body, mind and spirit. Saying 'no' to treatments, operations, medications or investigations that are not adequate for a particular person, or are not wanted or not needed, have repercussions at personal, local, national and global levels. Small movements lead to larger ones; small acorns grow into oaks. The listening and sharing we do is cumulative. Anything that one person does can help another by example.

Clearly, I am not saying that treatments, operations, medications or investigations should not be given or taken. I am, however, saying that we cannot live beyond our means any longer, and therefore decisions of how and how much depends on many variables, the most important of which is the person involved and his or her understanding of need and personal responsibility. Saying 'no' can be very difficult, but it can also be very liberating (see the discussion on strike action in Chapter 7).

In a class of students for a (postregistration) Bachelor of Science programme, I asked some questions relating to saying 'no'. I asked the students how many of them would accept organ transplants for themselves: only a few would. Asked if they would recommend organ transplants for their relatives, about the same number said that they would. When I asked them about blood transfusions, half the class said that they would not want them. Their reasons for their decisions were varied: they wanted 'bodily integrity'; they did not want to remain on medication for the rest of their lives; they knew too much of the process of organ harvesting to feel comfortable about it.

While it is possible to say that such arguments can only be made by 'insiders', it is precisely such arguments that also need to be debated and known about by those who will eventually benefit (or otherwise) from the results. When patients say, 'I wish I had known', it is too late to undo the damage. We need to help people individually and society at large to say less often, 'I wish I had known.' The task of saying 'no' and helping others to say 'no' is vast but also becoming easier.

The creative 'no' is not a 'no' for a purpose or an end other than being creative. It is not a 'no' in order to save money or even to further altruistic causes. The creative 'no' is creative in itself and is therefore liberating and empowering. The power thus given and taken is also creative as it enables people to see and treat each other as brothers and sisters rather than as experts and lay people, or those who give and those who take. When people are empowered, they become enabled to work with their own subconscious and unconscious parts (in the archetypes). Saying 'no' enables us to say 'yes'.

Saying 'yes' in nursing

Opposites need to balance each other, and, when they do, they are no longer opposites but part of the same essential whole. When we are able to say 'no' to games of power and control, we become able to say 'yes' to sharing, engaging in dialogue and actions that enhance relationships and personalities.

Saying 'yes' in nursing is therefore the activating force to share the 'mountain of experience' described in Chapter 1. We need to share our knowledge and skill not only with our clients and patients, but also, ever more clearly and urgently, with all those who are in positions of management and government at local, national and international levels. Unless we share and speak our truth, we will simply be forgotten. This does not mean that we have to shout louder than others or make ourselves more important than others; it means making sure that we are heard equally with others. It is in the sharing that we can advance. The old adage of 'it is in sharing that we receive' – in giving away that we gain – comes into its own in this argument.

One clear area where health professionals say 'yes' or 'no', as the case may be, is when they take industrial action. Such action is directed at management or at government rather than at patients and clients, so it carries a different weight. This topic will be addressed in more detail in Chapter 7.

Johnson (1977, p. 63) makes the point that saying 'no' comes late in a woman's psychological development and may only have to be spoken occasionally. The task that comes before is that of learning to be generous. The need in women to say 'yes' in order to feel accepted and fulfilled has to be transcended every now and again with the creative 'no'. However, generosity has to be there, otherwise the 'no' does not work and is not creative. I have been using these tasks as metaphors for what is happening in nursing, and so, to finish this discussion, I want to highlight a few links that have been made.

The 'mountain of experience' represents this generous aspect of the feminine psyche well. It is there, and we need to share it and have done so already. The creative 'no', however, may now represent something like saying, 'I will give of my knowledge and experience, but not on any terms. I will be generous and will share of myself and my knowledge and expect you to do the same. When we do this, we are not only equal, but also enhance each other's humanity, thus becoming full partners and colleagues'. This is not a simple thing to say and is certainly not a simple thing to accept in a world where inequality still often rules. We no longer accept that we should feel privileged to be invited to take part in debates and decisions: it is our right and our duty.

Only when we are aware of the power of our 'no' and our 'yes' can they become creative words and actions. This means being aware of the power of the words when they are not used creatively. The shadow and the archetype are never far away from us and they have been frightening us, and holding us in their grip and thus disabling us for a very long time. We cannot get rid of them or dismiss them as fantasy, but we need to acknowledge and accept them and work with them. By accepting the conscious and the unconscious aspects of this 'personality' that is nursing, we can move forward.

There are books and articles without number written on the subject of moving nursing into a better position, one of more autonomy and power. Equally as much is said and written on being effective, practical, evidence-based or whatever the buzzword of the moment is. All of this is valid and good, but if those who make these claims and pronouncements do not take into account the collective unconscious force of these archetypal elements, they can never help to change the face of nursing, and the disillusionment will not go away. We have to take very seriously the power of saying 'no' to exploitation of every kind – at a personal, professional, social, economic, environmental, medical, scientific, technological, spiritual, political and global level. Only when nurses have found their means of saying 'no' in a creative way whenever they meet it, will people respect their 'yes' in a different light and nurses will be able to give it generously.

6

The Ethical is the Visionary

If we want to see more of the good news than the bad we will have to do it for ourselves. It is no good waiting for some unidentified 'they' to fix our world for us. (Handy, 1997, p. 260)

It is a fact that nurses and nursing have for a long time waited for some knight in shining armour to 'fix it' for them. Because this knight has never turned up, nurses have become disillusioned with their vision and their reality. When nurses can understand why fairy tales will not work, but that the real archetype of the nurse and the woman who can say both the creative 'yes' and 'no' is what matters, they will then be able to take their vision upon themselves again and make it work for themselves. The vision is one of equality with other health professionals, of relationships and community, of working and being able to work professionally in such a way as to use their creativity for the benefit of society as a whole.

Building on the groundwork of the foregoing chapters, the remaining chapters point more to future possibilities and ideals. Much of what I have written so far is only applicable when seen as the possible, and possibilities have to be based on solid principles.

'Visionary leadership' is one of the five values identified by the ICN in 1997 as being necessary to guide nurses and nursing into the next century. The other values ('guiding principles or ideals') are:

- inclusiveness
- flexibility
- partnership
- achievement.

When 'mission statements' became popular, it was often felt that, before a 'mission' could be formulated, a step back had to be taken to be clear what the 'vision' was in fact about. In this book, I have, in a sense, gone yet another step back and analysed what the vision is based on. The basis is an ethical stance that asserts that 'people matter' and that what they mind about matters. In order to understand this stance and make it a reality we need to be able to:

- dream the undreamed-of
- imagine the unimaginable
- envisage the unenvisaged
- think the unthinkable
- believe the impossible
- consider that which has never been considered before
- dare to go where others have not dared to go
- try what has not been tried before
- think big, wide, futuristically.

This is a tall order, but, if nursing is to survive, it is in fact no longer a tall order but basic ethical thinking and action.

Vision and visions

With the language of 'vision', we are into the other-worldly and the imaginary. I will therefore start with a story that is situated in both this world and that of the tale.

One day a Yogi met a Sufi poet.

In his wish to prove how well Yoga had worked for him and how good he was at it, the Yogi handed a sword to the Sufi with the instruction to strike him – the Yogi – hard with it. After some persuasion the poet did this and the sword bounced off the Yogi.

At the insistence of the Yogi, the poet struck again several times and each time the sword rebounded, leaving the Yogi unharmed.

In his turn, the Sufi then asked the Yogi to take back his sword and to be struck with it himself.

The Yogi, knowing that the poet was untrained in Yoga, was extremely reluctant to do this. However, he did as he was bidden. He brought the sword down on top of the Sufi's head, with which the sword passed cleanly through the Sufi, meeting no resistance, and came to rest on the ground, between his feet.

The Sufi smiled and, bowing to the Yogi, went his way.' (Irvine, 1995, p. 20)

This story is meant to convey the impact of the will, either resisting or surrendering. In this, it succeeds very well: each of the people concerned demonstrates how these aspects of the will come to the fore in crucial situations. Clearly, each person thought that his way was the correct one, but each learned from the other that the opposite can work just as effectively.

A different aspect of the will is perhaps more strongly demonstrated in this story. When an expert in one field believes that someone else is not as accomplished, clever or knowledgeable, he or she tends to mistrust the other person. We trust our own certainties, assumptions, knowledge, commitments, values, identities and philosophies (Rabbin, 1998, p. 23), and, in so doing, diminish the other person and do not take into consideration that this person may be just as expert – only in something else – equally as good and relevant. This is something of what has happened to nursing: 'experts' did not believe that nurses had what they had; therefore they would not put them to the test. Had they done so, they might have met something quite astonishing and utterly complementary to their own practice. More than ever now, nurses do and need to show and tell the world that they have extraordinary expertise of a different kind, one which is entirely complementary to what is already on offer.

A very different aspect of vision was considered by Gandhi. According to Meadows (1995, p. 13), Gandhi gave his grandson Arun a talisman on which were written 'seven blunders' that are the cause of violence in the world. These blunders are:

- wealth without work
- pleasure without conscience
- knowledge without character
- commerce without morality
- science without humanity
- worship without sacrifice
- politics without principles.

According to Meadows, Gandhi was not 'calling for work without wealth or humanity without science; he was calling for work *and* wealth. Science *and* humanity. Commerce *and* morality. Pleasure *and* conscience'.

Part of the vision that we have to recapture is this very basic truth that 'either/or' leads us nowhere but that 'and' is the operative word, the bridge, the vital element in all our dealings. Most of us play the 'yes, but...' game quite regularly: 'would so-and-so... help you?': 'yes, but...'. When we can learn to say, 'yes, and...' in such situations, we will have moved significantly. Navone (1977, p. 27) says that:

> all stories should begin with the word 'And'. ...this would remind us that no experience ever begins; there was always something that preceded it.

'And' is in the 'I *and* Thou' of relationships; in the 'yes *and* no' of psychological growth, and in the realisation that whatever we have said or understood, any story has more to it than what is obvious because the beginning and the end of it are not usually accessible. We can only work with the given present, which is why the tenet 'people matter' is so important.

The blunders to which Gandhi is pointing are not new. Perhaps every generation and culture has complained of similar effects. The only difference is that, today, we are more globally aware of the facts and their effects. I will return to these aspects throughout this chapter.

Nursing – at least in the UK – has been so hemmed in by tradition and hierarchies, and of late by bureaucracy and policies, that it now needs the sort of input that only a 'vision' can give it. Simply rearranging a few ideas here and there is not going to be sufficient. We have looked inwards for such a long time and so avidly bemoaned the fact that we have a lower status than other health professionals that it seems we need an explosion more than a vision to bring light on to the scene in order to make nursing viable. Such an explosion, however, has to come from within as only this will satisfy us as nurses and be acceptable in any real way. We need to find our own voice; this comes from hearing ourselves and being available enough to our own inner spirit to lead us to some 'visions'.

Here again, it may be not so much *either* an explosion *or* a vision, but both.

The vision (singular) is the ethical stance that 'people matter'. How we approach this basic truth may indicate the different visions (plural) that guide us from the point of view of culture, religion or other tradition.

Any kind of vision involves some dreaming, speculating and playing. It also involves being awake and available to the unexpected and the unknown. When we become too adult and lose our childlike sense of surprise, we may no longer be fit for visions. Children are not able to calculate in the same way as adults and therefore do not first see the dangers that their actions entail. When watching a child of perhaps two years old recently, I was astonished to see that, whenever he came to an obstacle, he simply rolled over it. His mother had a hard time trying to stop him by pointing out that he might get hurt. Of course, he did not get hurt because children rarely do at that age. To him, an obstacle was only there to exercise his body. Perhaps this is a little parable of what nursing can aspire to.

> In nursing and the world at large, we are beginning to have a new sense of the importance of visions, the spiritual aspects of life in general and the need for connecting again with the parts of ourselves that were neglected when the pursuit was only for the material. What we are finding, however, is that the known and familiar images and language of spirituality no longer fit easily, leading us to find our own ways of expressions and symbolism. Our visions are therefore also not entirely traditional; maybe we do not even recognise that what we have (had) is a vision.

Spiritual components

Visions are the possibilities of tomorrow, be they the practical or the spiritual kind. This is perhaps the problem: we use the word 'spiritual' and imagine that everybody uses the word in the same way or that we all know what we mean by it. Clearly, we do not.

'Spiritual' and 'religious' are not necessarily synonymous. Many people speak of a spiritual hunger, but they do not want anything to do with organised religion of whatever tradition. Someone who enjoys nature may be described as a spiritual person; conversely, we can think of very religious people (those who attend religious worship regularly) who would not be described as spiritual because their outward practices have led them to be insensitive to the needs of others.

The way in which spirituality is usually understood today is as relating to anything concerning the spirit. And spirit, it is often pointed out, is that which gives life to something or is the capacity to see something bigger or wider, in other words, that which makes something whole. We cannot see it or touch it, but, without spirit, much of what we do or how we relate is lifeless.

Sheldrake and Fox (1996, p. 74) are very clear that spirit and soul are not the same:

> Dualism is based on the notion that soul and spirit are the same thing. St Augustine said: 'Spirit is whatever is not matter'. He takes spirit entirely out of everything that's matter. Aquinas says that spirit is the vitality in every being, in all matter, including in our souls. So hopefully spirit is in soul. But not if our souls are dead or barely purring. That's the point. Body and soul are ours but spirit is not. We are body and soul but spirit is not ours; it's greater than our bodies and souls. ...We're not in control of spirit. Spirit is everyone's and no one's. No one possesses spirit. It's not private property. No church owns it and no religion owns it. It's greater than the soul. Spirit requires receptivity, and open heart, a letting go.

Sheldrake, a British scientist, and Fox, an American writer on creation spirituality, discuss science and spirituality in their book, which takes the form of a dialogue (1996). Sheldrake (p. 19) explains that the idea of nature as inanimate has been replaced by the idea of nature as organised into fields. Fox (p. 72) elaborates on this when he asks, 'What is a field? It is a space for playing in. A field is a place for running in, frolicking in, dreaming in, soaring in, stumbling in, investing our passions in. I think all of those are images of the soul.' In the words of these two authors, what people today are looking for is how to enlarge the human soul, or how 'to grow soul' (p. 72).

Fox (p. 73) traces through history how various writers have described the relationship of body and soul, and he concludes that people most in touch with their souls all say the same thing: 'the soul is not in the body but the body is in the soul'. He considers this to be a 'fundamental shift of consciousness'. 'Believing that our body is in our souls means our souls are as large as the world in which we live, as the fields in which our minds play, and as the field in which our hearts roam'. Taking this image further, Fox (p. 80) says:

> if our souls are all over the place, if we're projecting them out there all the time, what an incredible invitation to be responsible for taking care of our souls, so that we are projecting the best of ourselves: grace and blessing and not envy, resentment or hostility. In other words, our morality is not a private matter. It's totally public. We've been saying that the other creatures are grace-filled but that we can get less and less grace-filled through envy and other issues. This seems to me to be a new way of approaching morality. It's not about 'dos' and 'don'ts', but about filling up our spaces in order to respond to one another with blessing to blessing and with grace to grace.

In 1997, 'nursing guru' Stephen Wright caused a stir in UK nursing when he revealed why he had 'given up the bright lights, champagne and Armani suits'. He had 'hit on something infinitely more valuable' (Salvage, 1997, p. 28). He said that 'failure to explore the spiritual basis of nursing is, I believe, a major cause of the horrendous levels of demoralisation, burn-out, sickness, suicide and wastage' (Wright, 1997, p. 32). Wright and Salvage wrote in the *Nursing Times*, and, judging by the many letters printed in subsequent editions of the journal, they had struck a deep cord with readers. At the same time, a lengthy article in similar vein appeared in the Swiss nursing journal *Krankenpflege/Soins infirmiers* (El-Bakkali-Bellini, 1997, pp. 54–8).

Returning to the argument that nursing is paralysed and inactive because 'others' have not taken it seriously, it could now be said that the demoralisation is caused by envy, resentment and hostility. Wright is correct in pointing to the fact that nursing has not paid enough attention to its soul, but the collective 'soul' also needs attention.

The collective unconscious and the collective consciousness are, in these images of fields and projections, part of the archetype of the nurse (Chapter 4). The nurse who withholds care and treatment may do so as a result of being demoralised through resentment and envy. If, as Sheldrake and Fox (1996, p. 80) point out, morality is not a private matter but a totally public one, nurses have to act publicly if they are to act morally. This may mean making their resentment and envy very clear, as well as going beyond it by engaging with the problem in a positive way. Nurses have to speak. Only in this way can they enlarge their 'soul' – filling up their space with 'blessing and grace' – and enable the archetype or shadow of the nurse to be integrated. Rather than letting the shadow of the nurse wreak havoc by extending the field of her soul ever more widely in destructive immorality, the use of the 'creative no' must come into its own here.

'Playing' seems to be a very important aspect of any life. We are 're-created' when we 'play' rather than when we strain every muscle or grey cell to get something accomplished. To act ethically, we have not only to act rightly, but also to create the spaces in which the soul can grow, flourish and be nourished. By saying that 'the ethical is the visionary', I am saying that it is ethically as important to develop our 'visions' as it is to decide rightly. The spiritual aspect of life cannot be overlooked and indeed dare not be overlooked, otherwise we harm ourselves and our morality.

A conference speaker asked his audience if they had ever thought what would be the first question that God would ask of them when they got to heaven. The speaker's emphatic answer to his own question was that God would ask, 'Have you had fun?' Maybe he has a point.

When we take the idea on board that the soul is larger than the body and surrounds it, we are immediately much more aware of other people's souls. Our first contact with other people is a 'soul contact' more than a 'body contact'. Some people have always known this and can describe 'auras'. Not everyone is gifted in this way, and we do not need to be so to realise that any contact with another person is a 'holy' contact and every person is a 'Thou'. We do not need to use religious language for this because the idea that 'people matter' is good enough and important enough in itself. Those of us who may feel awkward about talking of 'spiritual' things with clients and patients may feel encouraged that nurses do not have to talk of anything special. Simply being aware that we meet naturally as more than bodies says enough.

These ideas can take us into visions of which we had never dreamt. Because they concern us as people generally, and not just as individuals, they are ethical.

Imagination

According to the poet Mary Shelley, 'the great instrument of moral good is the imagination' (*Oxford Dictionary of Quotations*, 1993). It seems again and again to be imagination rather than invention that leads the world forward in substantive ways. Apparently, when NASA, the US Space Agency, first considered landing a craft on the moon, they invited a number of scientists to come together for a while and imagine ('play') how this might work in practice. In this way evolved the idea of the lunar buggy.

In 1980, Rogers (p. 200) wrote that 'our schools, our government, our businesses and corporations are permeated with the view that neither the individual nor the group is trustworthy'. Many of the religions of the world start with the basic principle that people are sinful and in need of control. It takes little imagination to transfer this to nursing and the need for the hierarchy that has dominated it so strongly for so long. Those who are so dominated eventually believe that they are 'sinful', worthless and in need of control. They come not only to believe, but also to accept, that this is their state. Young people who start their nursing education will, sooner or later, be aware that they have joined the profession when they identify with this culture, because then they have been 'baptised' into it. The religious language is not inappropriate, but a medical one can also be used. At the point at which nurses have acquired the disease called 'nursing culture', they are able to pass it on to the next generation like an inherited genetic disorder.

Yet Rogers' experience showed him that another paradigm is possible:

given a suitable psychological climate, humankind is trustworthy, creative, self-motivated, powerful and constructive – capable of releasing undreamed-of potentialities. (Rogers, 1980, p. 201)

These undreamed-of potentialities must be and are part of the imagination that is inherent in all of us. What is needed is the 'psychological climate'.

Wolinsky (1994, p. 5) says something similar in explaining the theory of chaos:

by attempting to manage the chaos, or apparent randomness of the world, we have created separate subjective structures and internal universes to explain such things. Unfortunately, creating structures to manage or explain chaos *continues* the chaos. It is through *allowing* chaos that higher orders can be revealed.

When the climate or *milieu* is favourable, anything can happen; the astonishing thing is that it tends to be 'good'. When people are not controlled by others who are afraid of losing control, the power they use is a positive one.

Necessity leads us to invent and create many objects and ideas, but if our imagination is only borne out of necessity, we have not yet developed the child within which is free and creative. It is perhaps a sign of the times that most of us, indeed, have to learn to recognise this child again when we are adult. I have always found it significant that the Bible presents us with the image of our 'parents' as having arrived fully grown. In psychological terms, Adam and Eve had to learn to be children. Indeed, the story of the serpent and the apple seems to be a story of their having to learn to 'play' with such images in their lives, and this may be a metaphor that we have to do likewise. When we regain the capacity to be childlike, we can be morally creative.

Part of the capacity for imagination is the need to listen: to ourselves, to the environment, to other people. Above all, it is a listening to our own inner self. This 'inner' self is not something located inside us, not even in our brains. If our souls are all around us, the 'inner' is confined not to our bodies but to the experience of all things. This enables us to listen to people, events and objects in ways which may be quite new, allowing them to address us by ways and means that we might not have realised before. This gives us the capacity to imagine.

Below, I will consider in particular the aspect of leadership
in this visionary context, but here I want to address other points
specifically related to nursing in the area of the imagination.

In April 1994, the DoH issued the report *The Challenges for
Nursing and Midwifery in the 21st Century* (the 'Heathrow Debate').
This is an interesting document as it has a feeling of 'play'
about it in the sense of active imagination having been at work
during the debate and the writing of the report. A few highlights from the text can give a flavour:

New opportunities and changing attitudes will pose new ethical
challenges for society. (p. 3)

Current distinctions between health services and social services will
have blurred [by 2010]. (p. 6)

A set of assumptions – 'benchmarks' – will operate by 2002, constituting a framework which becomes 'a field for discussion defined
by two dimensions: length... and... breadth. But to draw out some
of the strategic issues for nursing requires looking from a third
dimension. (p. 6)

[Care is seen] as a process of human interaction, not as mechan-
ical repairs. (p. 11)

There will be a smaller place for control by professionals, and a
much greater need for empathy and imagination. (p. 14)

Now the spotlight is on effectiveness, and how much the practitioner *achieves*. The new perceptions are extending the concept of
accountability beyond narrow professional issues. (p. 15)

Ethical dilemmas and conflict over priorities may become more open.
(p. 15)

Training programmes need to start from the assumption that they
are serving a learning organisation, and explicitly embody an evolu-
tionary approach. (p. 18)

the unity of nursing will need nurturing. (p. 21)

the 'era' of health care is over, changing to one of health promotion. A view that recognises that perfect health does not exist, that
people's *quality* of life is the key variable, is more in tune with the
nurse's perception. Nurses believe that their own insight should be
available at all levels – for the patient, for the local community and
where commissioning and policy decisions are taken. (p. 23)

This selection of topics and ideas shows what imagination and realistic guesswork can create. Within these possibilities, the individual's own imagination has to be applied and tried. While it may be relatively easy for a group of high-powered bureaucrats to think and write such a report, these ideas have to be made to work in specific situations. This is where the crunch comes and the obstacles begin to appear. With enough support, however, it should be possible; the real question is if this support is really there. It may be this which takes the most imagination yet: to dare to support colleagues in such a way that they can act morally, ethically, empathetically, professionally and effectively.

The future of health care is not like the past albeit faster and more technical. The future will be very different in style, approach and technique. The task for nurses so far has been largely to adapt to the given circumstances and events. It must be said that nurses have been very successful at this but, as I showed in Chapter 1, nurses have not been given the recognition due to them or have not been taken seriously as pioneers. The ethical task and responsibility of nurses in and for the future will be not only to react quickly to changes, but also to anticipate the changes, to *imagine* the future and thus to *create* the future in such a way that it will be one in which 'people matter' – nurses themselves and their clients and patients.

The DoH (1994, p. 6) report envisaged that, by the year 2002, '80% of surgical interventions will be by minimal access; 60% of surgery will be day case; acute hospital beds in District General Hospitals will be reduced by at least 40%'. This may have been too radical a vision, but without such imagination, we will never see further than the tip of our noses.

Nurses must be inventive and imaginative at every level (the following list deliberately not being in any hierarchical order):

- in nursing education, which needs to be ongoing (UKCC, 1992b, p. 9)
- in direct 'hands-on' care (Griffiths, 1997)
- in preventive health care
- in community-centred developments (Smith, 1997, p. 107)
- in issues of human rights

- in disseminating information and raising awareness of health issues in schools, industry, businesses, commerce and non-governmental organisations
- in being concerned with issues that indirectly impact on health, such as farming, transport, genetic manipulation, the environment, employment and unemployment, housing and waste
- in local, national and international government (Glover, 1998, p. 17)
- in following trends and strategies, and considering their implications for nurses
- in experimenting with flexible roles (Langstaff and Gray, 1997).

The possibilities for imagination and vision are endless. It frequently takes little more than a certain curiosity or permission to look at an issue sideways or after taking a step backwards and achieving a greater distance.

Gough (1998, p. 26) wonders how often nurses find themselves struggling to implement a policy that makes no sense to their ways of working and thinking. She states that:

> the health reforms of the past decade provide a stunning case study of the marginalisation of the nursing contribution. In 1984 the restructuring of the health service and the introduction of general management decimated the, albeit embryonic, nursing management structure. Nurses lost their seats on the executive decision-making bodies in the NHS. They were replaced by general managers, some of whom were nurses but many who may not have understood the notion of skilled nursing care.

Gough goes on to cite many more examples of where nurses have been sidelined but then mentions one particular 'coup' that nurses have achieved: the changes made to the NHS (Primary Care) Bill in the light of concerted lobbying. Gough also advocates that groups of nurses can achieve more than single individuals.

Groups of people undoubtedly have more impact, but such actions start with a single 'vision' or an idea that is imaginative. What this points to is that we need to talk and share such ideas and visions. The time is really over when we each just did our job in our own corner. Unless we talk, others will not hear of our ideas and cannot develop their own imagination. Ethics is always about what happens between people, and the ethical stance may therefore be to share these ideas. Yes, nursing has been marginalised and disregarded, and much of it is our own fault for not having shared and talked and fought. The past cannot be undone so the ethical stance – which is always concerned with the potentially possible – is to consider the present and run with the imagination of what could be.

I will return to some of these topics in the last chapter.

Leadership

Senge (1990, pp. 359–60) makes some interesting statements about leadership. His book is about learning disciplines and what he calls 'learning organisations'. Leaders of such organisations, he suggests, have the ability:

> to develop conceptual and communication skills, to reflect on personal values and to align personal behavior with values, to learn how to listen and to appreciate others and others' ideas. ...They provide a framework for focusing the effort to develop the capacity to lead. Systems thinking, personal mastery, mental models, building shared vision, and team learning – these might just as well be called the *leadership disciplines* as the learning disciplines. ...Ultimately, people follow people who believe in something and have the abilities to achieve results in the service of those beliefs. Or, to put it another way, who are the natural leaders of learning organizations? They are the learners.

What Senge points to so clearly is that those who lead must first of all be able to learn. This is not simply learning facts but learning from each other and with each other. In this way, all the people together are and become leaders. Or, to put it in the language that I have used earlier, sharing is one of the important elements of all living.

Taking up an other point I made, Antrobus (1998, p. 66) says that nursing leaders need to develop skills to do the following (emphasis added):

- Influence both nursing practice *and* health policy
- Create a language that spans both nursing *and* management
- Scan for changes in the environment *and* think strategically.

Leaders seem to be people who can span ideas *and* actions, leading *and* learning, giving *and* taking. In other words, they are the people who can 'embody' for the group or the organisation the fact that there are no polar opposites but that 'everything is made of the same essential substance' (Wolinsky, 1994, p. 109). These ideas are essential in quantum theories, and Wolinsky points out that it is only our minds that have divided opposites and created pairs of opposites. Once we realise that there is no division, we see that it is 'only the label and the boundary which say they are not'. A leader is therefore someone who is able to recognise and create integrity at the practical and the psychological level. A leader is not someone who stands at the front and shouts, 'Follow me', but someone who can see more than just one side. Such a person needs to have a wide vision, a comprehensive language and a soul that can touch and feel the souls of many different people, ideas and objects.

We are all leaders of others, however inadequately we do it. Parents are leaders of their children, student nurses lead those younger than themselves, and ward managers lead a varied team of qualified and non-qualified staff. Not everyone wants to be in a position of obvious leadership, and this needs to be respected. However, leaders are not only born, but also made, in particular by others who recognise in them certain qualities. According to the RCN (1996, p. 3):

Nurses who have the potential for development, in addition to a belief in nursing and empathy for people, may exhibit some of the following:

- a desire to influence (sometimes they may be angry)
- the ability to facilitate and enthuse others
- self-motivation
- working in a supportive style
- using authority with discretion
- acting with bravery and taking risks
- saying 'no'
- recognising their own limitations
- acting with confidence
- allowing others to take the praise.

Garbett (1998, p. 68) catalogues 'an alarming array of concerns' that the chief nurses of various trusts had mentioned in a survey. They were worried about 'how ill-defined their jobs were, how unable they felt to make a difference and how they felt nursing was not valued in their organisation'. The greatest influence on these managers on their job satisfaction was their relationship with the chief executive. However, many of them seemed to stay in their post for only a relatively short time, their salaries being an important element in this.

These findings point to the real difficulties of 'life at the top'. No job, not even a 'new' post, starts completely from scratch. The history of the institution, the idea and the people involved cannot be overlooked. A 'new broom' may sweep cleaner than an old one, but the emphasis in management is on people rather than brooms. That may often be the problem: a 'package' is offered, or an idea, concern or problem is in need of a solution, and there may be no solution because the human element is not taken into consideration. When we concentrate on a problem, we become part of the problem. It is only when we can concentrate on goals that we become part of the goal. The people at the top may easily become part of 'the problem' of the whole organisation – because they have to deal with, and hopefully solve, so many actual problems – so that they become too disabled and impotent to make any real difference. Not until they can step sideways can they be creative.

A problem arising directly from this situation for nurse managers may be that they become so busy that they have little time to meet with peers from other organisations, or even their own, to play, imagine and 'freely associate' with each other. They become more and more isolated, and, in order to 'save their souls', have to withdraw and find another job. They cannot therefore make the environment in their own organisation one in which human activity and living are conducive to health and healing. The pressure is on production and getting the bottom line right. What is missing is the 'organic and fuzzy and warm and cuddly and mysterious' (Dennett, 1984, p. 1453) of wholeness and relationships. The point made by Antrobus (1998) is that managers are the people who understand above all the '*and*' or bridge from one environment to

another. It is clearly this which they have to practise for themselves and for their own colleagues. For this to happen, they
need a good dose of 'proper selfishness'.

I am reminded here of a little book (Türcke, 1997, p. 1)
showing on its front cover a drawing made in 1928. The picture
shows:

> Christ on the cross with gas mask and army boots; the cross beam
> broken off at both ends; Christ's left hand, which this releases,
> holding high a little cross; the whole picture signed 'keep your mouth
> shut and go on serving'. The real Christ on the cross uttered that
> terrible cry, 'My God, my God, why have you forsaken me?

The picture shows him with a gas mask on so he cannot shout.
I expect that many managers' experience is also one of having
been forgotten and forsaken. Their way of keeping going is
keeping their mouths shut and going on serving because there
is no alternative. One may need to ask who put the gas mask
on their face and why. One may also need to ask why managers
consent to having gas masks put on their faces.

Leaders are often expected to be 'saviours', but systems that
need such figures have to consider why they need saviours in
the first place. Saviours have an impossible job if they allow
themselves to be used in that role. However, if they do not play
the role, they too are ousted. Saviours and rescuers can only
fulfil their role by turning the system upside down and start by
listening and empowering the 'little' people. They, and not those
who can look after themselves, are the ones who need rescuing.

It is only in times of crises that we tend to want strong and
charismatic leaders. The history of the 20th century should show
us, however, how dangerous such leaders and such needs are.
Learning to live with uncertainty, ambiguity and complex situations must be a more creative way. This requires not just one
leader but a team of people who can lead and learn together,
thus enabling all to take a leading role in such deliberations.

Another religious image may be appropriate. The rise of the
Reformation in the Middle Ages split the Christian Church
down the middle, but it also gave it wholly new vistas. One of
those new aspects was 'the priesthood of all believers'. This
gave people a new commitment and encouraged personal
responsibility. The concept is not disputed today by any branch

of the Church, although the interpretation of it necessarily involves stressing different aspects.

> In an age of enormous change, specially in health care, the image could be stretched to 'the leadership of all health care personnel'. This does not detract from the specific leadership of some people, but, being aware of our own responsibility as leaders, this idea enhances the self-image and confidence of those nurses who at present feel belittled and unimportant.

One problem for leaders is that, the higher they get in the hierarchy, the more diffuse become their responsibilities. While this is desirable for giving more scope and encouraging an approach that tends to be responsible and proactive (Harwood, 1997, p. 66), it can also be very frustrating for people who have grown up with clear boundaries. The imagination – the proactive stance – can be scary and too much of a licence. When people at the top become too lonely, they may have to consider their situation again. When they lose their ability to imagine and envision, and play with ideas and dreams, they are in danger of producing the same in others by manipulating them and silencing them. Any idea of ethical behaviour then goes out of the window. In such circumstances, not only does one person behave unethically, but also the whole institution becomes unethical:

> Institutions have ethical lives and characters just as their individual members do. Health care organizations must look critically at how professed institutional values can best be realized in day-to-day interactions within the institution and with the wider community. ...Without a genuine humaneness pervading the activities and personnel of health care organizations, their mission of service to the sick is compromised. (Reiser, 1994, pp. 28, 35)

The job of leaders is supremely to address these points and ensure that they are recognised and met. More than ever these days, we need visionary leaders who are not remote figures. They may not:

stand out in a crowd; ...they (may) not mesmerize an attending audience with their brilliance or eloquence. Rather, what distinguishes them is the clarity and persuasiveness of their ideas, the depth of the commitment, and their openness to continually learning more. They do not 'have the answer'. But they do instil confidence in those around them that, together 'we can learn whatever we need to learn in order to achieve the results we truly desire'. (Senge, 1990, p. 359)

Such leaders make it possible for others to act ethically, so the ethical becomes the visionary and the visionary in turn is the ethical. These people enable others to mind about what matters to them, and this will lead all of them to say their creative 'no' and 'yes' appropriately. When the visionary is also the spiritual, 'no' is the necessary response to anything that stifles and reduces the human soul.

Visionary action

When we concentrate too hard on results and effectiveness, we are in danger of losing the creative aspect of living. We need to balance everything we do with the possibility of its being different and 'other'. Only in this way can our morality be maintained and our ethics be workable.

The vision must become the mission. Particularly in the UK, with the NHS celebrating its fiftieth anniversary of existence, it is impossible not to speculate what the next 50 years will bring. Gough (1998, pp. 30–2) makes the point that:

the capacity of nursing to care extends also to shaping the determinants of health that lie beyond the biological destiny or immediate physical environment of a person.

She sees societal health and community developments as part of nursing, which will also centre more on healing than on technical interventions. She ends her article by saying that:

we must trust that nursing can rediscover its confidence to turn the rhetoric of... white papers into a bright future.

Reading this leaves me with a strange sense of wishing for something that we somehow know we will never *really* get.

My response is that we do have that confidence because, I believe, the principle that 'people matter' is not something that we must first dig out or unravel. We have been working with it and can claim it and run with it. I hope that I am simply pointing to a few ideas of how it can be applied. Chapter 9 will highlight a few more visions.

7

The Ethical is the Political

Nurses always say that they went into nursing to care for people; if they had wanted to be political, they would have gone into politics.

We cannot care for another person – holistically or otherwise – without being aware of constraints, policies, injustice, inadequate resources, bad communication and inabilities to care effectively resulting from traditions and hierarchies. If we want to care holistically – and who does not? – we need not only to moan and grumble about these restraints, but also to do something about them. Restraints to good care are not only local and temporary: they have always existed, and they exist in every sphere of care. Moves to expand and extend roles, introduce 'supernurses', give titles and awards, and formulate the registration and regulation of nursing are political as much as professional moves. It is simplistic to say 'We want to care' yet be oblivious of our surroundings. If we do this, we show that we have not yet understood what care is, or is about. Or maybe we have not yet heard our own inner voice that cries out for justice, acknowledgement and being heard.

The inner voice does not say, 'I want to be a nurse because I want to be an angel.' Those who want to be angels presumably die and try to function from another dimension. If nursing is to be effective, it has to live, and live vigorously.

The word 'political' is for many people a slightly dirty word. It is connected with dealing in dark rooms, manoeuvring and the use of power for one's own advantages. I want to use the word in a much wider sense. By 'being political' I mean an awareness of the surroundings and influences on care and the ability to interact with them effectively. We do this all the time, but very often we do it surreptitiously, grudgingly and perhaps always with the feeling that we cannot win anyway whatever we do. We feel at the mercy of so many hostile powers and influences. When we allow ourselves to see them as friends rather than enemies, they can begin to work for us – and we with them.

One of the main issues in any debate on ethics and politics is justice.

Justice

Justice as a principle to hold society together is as old as the hills. During an early phase of development, all children are obsessed with the idea of 'fairness'. Later on, we learn that many things are not fair in life. However, by 'justice' I do not mean a simple equation with everybody having to have the same. Aristotle was concerned that 'equals should be treated equally and unequals unequally in proportion to the relevant inequalities' (Gillon, 1986, pp. 87–8). What the relevant inequalities are has to be interpreted, however, and herein lies the difficulty.

I have written elsewhere (Tschudin, 1992, 1994) on the ethical principle of justice and how it applies to nursing, and many other authors have done so more elaborately. My concern here is to highlight justice as an aspect of the political work of nurses to make themselves and their cause more relevant and appropriate. (Nor am I concerned with 'justice' in opposition to 'care' in the debate between Kohlberg and Gilligan. This is well treated in Kuhse, 1997, pp. 90–141.)

Puls (1993, p. 82) says:

> No issue raises the question of justice more immediately than that of food. Whose food is it that we line up for, bargain over, import and export, stockpile, and waste? Is not the ownership of food a fundamental question in our present world? Or the ownership of land of all the earth's resources, even of sunshine and rain?

Food is the one thing we all depend on, and nurses everywhere are concerned with it, but how much concerned with it are we really? When the bovine spongiform encephalopathy

(BSE) crisis blew up in Britain in 1996, Hunt (1996, p. 266) contacted 'three major UK organizations of professions allied to medicine' to enquire how far they had debated the issue. The outcome was perhaps not surprising: the RCN said that this subject had 'yet to be debated'; the Health Visitors' Association 'had received expressions of concern from its members' and had contacted the Ministry of Agriculture, Fisheries and Food; the Royal College of Midwives (RCM) 'revealed that there has been no thought given to the implications of BSE'. The crisis was over eating contaminated beef, which may lead to the crippling Creutzfeld-Jakob Disease. Why were nursing and midwifery organisations not more involved? More drastically, however, the vast number of nurses and health care professionals the world over live and work in areas where providing food is a daily struggle for survival. It is not enough that courageous nurses from wealthy countries go and work in drought-stricken countries; as a profession, we need to challenge why such droughts still happen.

Carlisle (1998, pp. 40–1) quotes nurse Geoffrey Prescott, who has worked with Médecins Sans Frontières, and sees his work linked to human rights:

> for example, we have a concept of emergency public health. In a state of emergency, you need six things to survive: clean water and basic sanitation; basic curative and preventive health care; shelter; clothes; basic nutrition; and safety and security. The first five are easy to see as medical needs. Safety and security are the things that would not occur immediately to a nurse.

In a statement worthy of being written in capital letters, and applying to nursing everywhere like a motto, Prescott says:

> Nurses provide the link between the people on the ground and the people who can change things.

If this is a possibility for nurses in areas of extreme difficulty, it should also be possible in more favourable circumstances. What this points to is the issue of human rights: how unequals are treated unequally. Chinombo (1998, pp. 81–4) describes how community health nurses in Malawi were instrumental in helping communities to solve their own health problems by supporting and empowering local people. When people were able to identify their own health problems, they could devise strategies to control them. She says, however, that:

> when programmes are limited due to lack of money, the government should try to support these community efforts in its budget.
> ...Failure to support communities will reduce their ability to achieve the desired health outcomes.

This last sentence points to the crux of any political action: if politicians, managers and leaders of all types want something achieved, they need to support it in the right way. If what they want is not beneficent, they must be challenged.

For nurses – people who 'nourish' and 'nurture' – food is perhaps only the most obvious example for making the point about justice. Justice relates to every sphere and action in health care. As nurses, we cannot overlook the injustices that go on throughout the world with regard to food: the miles that food travels around the world, putting local growers out of business; the water that such food needs to grow, leaving little water for the people growing the food, thus increasing the possibility of disease; the chemicals used on such foods because they grow in hostile climates, exposing people to toxic substances; the low wages that many people are paid for such 'dangerous' work; the profits that shareholders and the bosses of large companies and conglomerates such as Monsanto, rather than the people growing the food, earn and the genetic manipulation of foods, which will essentially only serve the conglomerates and potentially expose the whole population to unknown and as yet unimaginable risks.

These concerns are often viewed with a sense of helplessness: what can one person do in the face of blatant injustice thousands of miles from here? Paul (1998, p. 14) makes the point that:

> human rights instruments have hitherto always been written in terms of the individual versus the state. However, many of our future struggles for self-determination are likely to involve the people versus the corporation.

This is quite clearly also the increasing experience of nurses in this country. One person against the institution is likely to be dismissed, but a group of people cannot be dismissed so easily. Additionally, while the institution was limited to a hospital or a district, the impact of group action might have been impressive; when the organisation is impressively large, any protest needs to match it in comparison. This is far from easy, but neither should large organisations be able to overrule their employees and disregard those, however few, who make their concerns known. If they do, justice is not served.

Stories are often told of patients leaving hospitals malnourished, nurses putting food in front of patients who are unable to reach it, or patients being fed so quickly or disinterestedly that they cannot eat either enough or well enough. Such issues concern justice. Why is there either not enough food or not the right food available? Why are patients and clients neglected and simply not respected? When any kind of investigation goes on in the health services and elsewhere, a hunt normally starts for the person who has done the deed wrongly. This is inevitably the person at the end of the line. When we have hunted down this person, we feel justified. We forget, however, that any care happens only within a setting and a system in which such things are either tolerated or at least not challenged. It is not the person who is most at fault but the system, the organisation. It is there that we must look for justice.

As individuals and as a profession, we can no longer let such issues go by unchallenged. We owe it to ourselves and to the profession to take a stand in the face of injustice. We need to say 'no' more often and more clearly. We recognise issues of injustice only when we listen to our own needs for ethical behaviour and action, and this we learn only in contact with people who are clients, patients and colleagues. People matter – we matter – and what we mind about matters. It matters that we can say what matters to us and what we mind about. Paul (1998) points to the fact that large organisations are slowly but surely replacing governments in the power they wield, and, as nurses, we are part of organisations more immediately and directly than we are of governments and states. We cannot ignore what we are part of because the organisation pays us. This is clearly the crunch: we could be fired, but we also have power in the organisation, and the right use of power is the most obvious way of acting ethically. Both we and the organisation have to do right and uphold human rights: people matter.

Political awareness

At the beginning of 1997 – the year of the Labour Party's return to government in the UK after nearly 20 years of Conservative rule – Castledine (1997b, p. 58) pointed out that 'political activity means influencing for the purpose of allocating scarce resources wisely'. This is surely too narrow a view of political activity. When Labour was in opposition, Tony Blair (who became Prime Minister in 1997) made speeches that regularly featured 'sound-bites' promising that nurses could nurse again rather than filling out forms. In this, the 'new language of social justice' would be applicable, with Labour showing the way to 'what is just and unjust, fair and unfair, right and wrong' (Blair, 1996, p. 30). Can governments really be that black and white? And if they could, would this be desirable?

Jacobs (1996, p. 1) says, that:

the country [Britain] seems to be drifting aimlessly into the 21st century. The body politic frequently seems rudderless, swinging to and fro on passing waves, mesmerised by the smallest movements. The deep ocean currents of global change meanwhile move us powerfully and unnoticed underneath.

Every government promises to change this state of affairs, but, once in power, they find that it is much more difficult because of the number of interlinking wheels, which turn very slowly.

It is indeed a puzzling paradox that 'despite stunning achievements and more extensive efforts in health care, the level of disease in our society is escalating' (Goudzwaard and de Lange, 1995, p. 5). The Public Health Alliance (in Jacobs, 1996, p. 71) says:

Health is a fundamental good. Its promotion should be the aim of government policy. But this requires changes not just to health policy, but to the very idea of economic development itself.

Giddens (1997, p. 136) points to environmental factors that:

are probably coming more and more to influence patterns of health and illness. Pollution of the air, for example, may affect the health of thousands, or millions, of people. It follows that health care in the future should concentrate on creating more favourable environmental conditions for people to live and work in.

Political awareness, for nurses, comprises all these areas and aspects of life and living, of individuals and society. 'The NHS has become a political battleground' (Castledine, 1997b, p. 58), and all nurses are, for better or for worse, on this ground. The 'battlegrounds' are clearly visible to anyone with even a passing knowledge of the daily lived reality, mentioning here only the most obvious:

- the chronic long-term care of older people
- the health care of ethnic minorities
- the care of people with mental illness in the community and institutions
- community care.

More specific issues are that:

- long waiting lists increase morbidity
- violence in A & E has social roots
- the increase in infectious diseases such as TB and MRSA have causes and effects that are potentially devastating for society generally
- health care 'by post code' is viewed as being most unjust
- technology to extend life at both ends is costly and has brought with it multitudes of moral, ethical and social problems
- unemployment causes morbidity.

Nurses hear of these facts in the news media and meet them in their daily lives and via their colleagues but, as Prescott (Carlisle, 1998, pp. 40–1) mentions, do not or cannot link them to the wider issues. Our working patterns and social constructs have taught us to think in pigeon-hole fashion: I do my thing and you do yours. When new ideas, such as holistic care, surface, we take them on as 'a good thing' without knowing or studying the implications or indeed the concept. Holistic care is not only concerned with the person of the patient or client and his or her immediate surroundings. A 'package' of care sounds promising, but, even before it can be delivered, the many strands and components of the immediate situation and the wider context have to be considered too. This may involve nurses in work that is not 'directly' care centred when looked at from a reductionist point of view but has everything to do with care when seen from the standpoint of 'total' care. As so often, it depends how one interprets the meaning of the words. In his short article, Castledine (1997b, p. 58) concedes that, in his early days of nursing, he thought that he as a nurse:

> should remain politically neutral. However, over the years [his] views have changed because of all the reforms that have been made to the NHS.

This must be the case for many nurses of his generation and younger. The ideal of 'caring' seemed superior to 'getting entangled' in the business of politics. History has proved us wrong. When we try to close our minds to our surroundings, we tend, sooner or later, to come unstuck.

New insights and awareness are not enough for action, but awareness is necessarily the first step. The second step is acknowledging the awareness and owning it. Political awareness is the first need; the second is realising that we can do something. This equates with the notion that people matter and what they care about matters:

- I/you matter
- my/your voice matters
- my/your values matter
- my/your responsibility matters
- my/your contribution matters
- my/your thoughts and feelings matter
- therefore what I mind about matters
- what is given matters; I/you may not have chosen it, but, because it is here, we need to respect it and address it.

In politics, it matters supremely how we see, think, feel and speak, in other words, how we communicate matters. To acknowledge this is the first step towards any kind of action or change of attitude. Political action here may even mean something as simple as acting on the principle that people matter, rejecting the idea that people

> can be used, taken advantage of or belittled. Any change
> starts with acknowledging a given fact; these may be the
> given facts here.

Professional development

Florence Nightingale opposed state registration for nurses but
not education. According to Bradshaw (1994, p. 142), 'it was
not registration itself to which Nightingale was opposed, but
the kind of registration proposed'. Because Nightingale
believed that:

> the quality of the nurse, and thus of the care she gave, depended
> on her moral character, her inner motivating principles... were the
> heart of good nursing. ...If this spirit was eroded, Nightingale
> argued, then the standard of nursing care would no longer be the
> highest that was possible to achieve, but rather the lowest that was
> considered acceptable.

Would Nightingale turn in her grave if she knew what is
happening today? Perhaps she would, but then she would not
have had the luxury of being part of the historical developments, as we have.

Ideas and practices have come and gone, each trying to be
more applicable, adept or effective. The nursing process,
nursing models, primary care, extended and expanded practice, Project 2000, reflective practice and the like have all
widened the horizon. Perhaps the most significant development in nursing generally has been the move into higher
education. This has given nurses not only a higher profile, but
also more confidence to stand side by side with their colleagues,
in particular doctors. However, the many ingrained problems
with and within nursing have not yet significantly shifted.

Flatt (1997, p. 24) points to 'three issues which health care
professionals must address before any kind of new professionalism can develop':

Communication between health care workers is notoriously bad. Many recent investigations have underlined failures in communication that have led to poor outcomes for ill people. The professions do not communicate well.

Interdisciplinary rivalry has been part of poor communication in nursing. There is also a rivalry that has existed for decades between doctors and nurses. The protection of territories has often been paramount.

Physicians have been inculcated from day one in their training with the thought that they are responsible for everything to do with health care. This has led them to believe that they also control everything – including the role of the nurse and the fate of patients.

These sentiments are very similar to what Chambliss (1996) (Chapter 1) highlights. Problems with communication and interdisciplinary rivalry sap the energy of nurses and doctors, and perpetuate problems rather than solve them. Professionalism is not advanced when energy is constantly diverted into sidelines that help nobody and potentially harm patients and clients.

In recent years, many of the debates about professionalism have been concerned with the expansion of the nurse's role. Advanced practices, such as intravenous drug and fluid administration, suturing, defibrillation and drug prescribing have become routine for certain nurses and in certain situations. Yet many nurses also ask themselves whether this is advancing *their* practice or merely reducing that of doctors. Scott (1996, p. 1028) sees such practices as delegation. The British Medical Association (BMA) had issued a policy statement on the delegation of medical procedures to non-medically qualified staff, to which Scott responded:

> To delegate, by definition, is to give or commit duties to another as agent or representative. Therefore, to delegate medical care to nurses means that nurses are acting as the agent or representative of the doctor in such circumstances where the doctor is unable or unwilling to be his/her own agent or representative. Given that the BMA sees this as advantageous, there can be no clearer statement that the BMA persists in seeing nurses and other health-care staff as merely an adjunct to the central role of the doctor.

Murray (1998, p. 65) thinks along similar lines when he suggests that new clinical roles, such as 'emergency nurse practitioners in A & E, laparoscopic nurse practitioners in surgery, and medical support nurses in acute and mental health' seem simply to 'tackle the issues surrounding the intended reduction in the hours of work of junior hospital doctors'. He is unclear whether such roles will benefit nursing practice and future career movements for individual nurses or whether the:

> profession will benefit in respect of developing a body of nursing knowledge from these roles which will help to inform and guide practice and contribute to nursing's credibility and profile.

The more subtle changes in nursing, at least in the UK, are however, not in the practice but in the thinking behind the practice and in the wording used to convey this. Perhaps in line with higher education, nurses consider now that they are educated rather than trained and that this education is ongoing rather than simply a one-off. The new roles are no longer considered to be 'extended practice' because extension concentrates on activities rather than on the importance of holistic nursing care (UKCC, 1992b, p. 8). If holistic care is the central theme, practice must remain dynamic and 'able readily and appropriately to adjust to meet changing care needs'. The UKCC (1992b, p. 9) goes on to make a very important statement about professionalism when it declares:

> In order to bring into proper focus the professional responsibility and consequent accountability of individual practitioners, it is the Council's principles for practice rather than certificates for tasks which should form the basis for adjustment to the scope of practice.

This sentiment confirms the ICN (1997) values of 'visionary leadership, inclusiveness, flexibility, partnership and achievement'. In this area of professional development, there will always be tensions and trials. If leadership is to be visionary, it has to allow for failure and for changes as the vision develops. The inclusiveness surely points to the need to work co-operatively with colleagues. We need urgently to develop professionally in partnership with our colleagues rather than in opposition to them (David and Hopkins, 1998). One sometimes gets the feeling that, when nursing achieves something, it is like a feat, to the surprise and astonishment of our professional colleagues. This makes it clear why joint education is vital as the basis for all professional development and also why partnership, rather than opposition and autonomy, are necessary. Too much fragmentation can too easily lead to patient confusion.

Flexibility also points to the need to be adaptable, and inclusiveness and achievement point to areas of work where nursing is uniquely qualified to make changes by making other professionals and the public generally aware of ways and means of maximising health.

These good and laudable values do, however, also have a flip or shadow side. Leadership can be misunderstood; inclusiveness can lead to exclusion; flexibility can be taken advantage of by others (Butler, 1998); partnership can take too long to develop and may be too elastic a concept; and achievement may never be reached because the bandwagon may have rolled on. Professionalism itself is difficult to define and more difficult still to measure. Advanced nursing practice is inevitably concerned with recognition, and this tends to mean complicated job titles and confusion for clients and patients. The archetype, or shadow, is an integral part of any concept or person, so we need to consider also the potential chaos that these values can wreak. Yet they are necessary precisely for their unruliness. In our enthusiasm for something good, we may completely forget the negative side that holds us back: the unwillingness to lead, to be flexible, to achieve and to be partners, and the weight at nursing's heels in wanting to be exclusive. We may not – indeed we should not – be able to overcome these aspects because they are necessary to remind us of our vulnerability. 'Inclusiveness' may point to the fact that we need to include the shadows of our profession and work with them for them to be useful and helpful to us.

In the debate on professionalism and professional development, we can easily forget the main purpose: clients and patients (Bagnall, 1997, p. 24). If we do this, we will have dug our own grave. The challenge is rather that we learn how to be professional practitioners, able to 'create a highly skilled workforce, equipped to meet changing health care needs' (Bagnall, 1997, p. 25), keep the debate alive and give holistic care. When we can juggle all the various demands and not succumb to any of them, we may indeed be getting our voice heard.

Chambliss (1996, p. 184), who is not a nurse, encourages nurses by saying that 'for nursing, the crucial task is... a matter of regaining confidence in its own validity'. 'If nurses want to be heard, they will have to speak with their own authority, based on their own experience and their own values.' Chambliss considers this to be an ethical approach. In this setting, as in much else, the ethical is the political. It would seem that, when nurses keep the focus most clearly on clients and patients, roles and practices can change flexibly. When we look at ourselves, we lose this focus and tend to get lost in hierarchies and job titles and with details. These are important and necessary, but they are of lower priority. When we remember that people matter, we cannot go far wrong. Then our practice and our ethic lead us to responsibility and accountability, which are the real hallmarks of professionalism. Perhaps what we need to keep in mind, however, is that professional development will always be more of a journey than a destination.

Professional regulation

Since 1997, the UKCC has been using the motto 'Protecting the public through professional standards'. With this statement, the UKCC aims to clarify to society its role of regulating the profession.

> Professional regulation is the means by which order, consistency, and control are brought to a profession and its practice. (Affara and Styles, 1993, p. 7)

The problem with all regulation will always be how to combine effective control with individual professional freedom. Indeed, Affara and Styles (1993, p. 18) say that 'the scope of nursing practice as defined by law is often more restrictive than the ability of nurses to perform and the public need for their services'. The next conundrum must also be how much should be imposed by laws and governments, and how much the profession should regulate itself. A profession will always be ahead of its rule books, creating tension between the possible and the impossible.

Styles (1989, p. 32), a former president of the ICN, considers specialisation in nursing to be a tool towards a new kind of empowerment. To this end, she thinks that integration is essential if the profession is to survive and advance, and that the conditions for orderly change and empowerment are 'legitimacy, homogeneity and unity'. The danger with focusing on specialisation and advanced practice is that the rest of the workforce is left behind. It is easy for government ministers to pick out an aspect, such as nurse prescribing or creating 'supernurses', and declare them as 'the pinnacles of nursing development' (Scott, 1998, p. 508), glossing over the many other aspects that need attention. Paternalism from doctors has so long dogged the profession that we need to be very careful of the paternalism from government interventions on regulation.

One of the basic elements that make regulation possible is a definition, in this case of nursing. As every nurse knows, this has always eluded us. However, in English, unlike many other languages, we have an advantage in that we have the word 'nursing'. The problem still exists because the scope and purpose of nursing are not simply co-terminus with the functions of a nurse. Any regulatory system has to contain elements of (Affara and Styles, 1993, pp. 122–3):

- The purposes of regulation
- The specifications of the administrative agent or body (powers, officers)
- The definitions of nursing and nurses
- Standards of education and practice
- Criteria for meeting these standards
- Administrative procedures for approving schools, licensing and registration, disciplinary procedures and so on
- Any special circumstances which might apply.

When South African nurses were considering how their new regulatory authority should function, and who or what should be its statutory home following the apartheid years, they made many of the changes based on Affara and Styles' (1993) work. The procedure was carried out in as truly a democratic way as is ever possible with a large population, giving all concerned a sense of involvement in their own regulation through postal questionnaires and meetings, and resulting in the creation of the Democratic Nurses Organisation of South Africa (Uys, 1996). Perhaps few nurses these days are in the privileged position of making choices concerning their statutory or regulatory body because most of them are in place. What nurses everywhere need to do is to keep these bodies relevant and accessible.

The regulatory body gives legitimacy to and is a safeguard for practice, but it can also become a burden on our backs, allowing us only to look at the ground on which we are standing. Being a professional practitioner calls us, however, to look at the far horizons – indeed the stars – and be visionary and innovative. If we want such a body to be our body, we must also encourage its officers to do the same. This may mean that those registered with such a body must on occasion 'push' it to be more up front and trend setting, or 'pull' it when it is not sufficiently flexible, partnership minded or inclusive. The body is setting standards for ethical care: the body itself must therefore act ethically. The responsibility of all of us nurses is to ensure this.

Such a body has to be accessible for nurses who may need help and guidance in difficult situations, and it also has to be supported by its users. The UKCC Council elections have not attracted great attention in recent years, and this is regrettable. If nursing is to be inclusive, the apathy thus displayed is unethical. There should not be a wide gap between them and us, between officers and ranks, policy makers and workers. If being ethical is being political, it should be much easier to have casual contact between the various aspects of the profession. All of us have to be visionary, flexible and creative about our practice, and that means being interested in what is happening in every sphere. Nurses have, for very long, suffered from the fact that policies and rules were made for us rather than by us; made by men for women; by politicians for nurses. If we want to change such practice and culture, we have to do it ourselves. We may not always know how to do it most easily, but we certainly know what we want done, what we want to be regulated and what needs to be left alone. Our mountain of experience is formidable.

Partnerships

The idea of partnership is becoming more and more important. Like so many ideas, it may need to be defined before it can be applied. It is certainly wider than simply thinking of close professional colleagues, such as doctors, physiotherapists, social workers and so on. Nurses have close partnerships with all who care for other people in any way. This may include agencies concerned with public health, probation, housing, immigration, informal caregivers and consumer representation, to mention only the most obvious. Nurses have regular contacts with police and with emergency crews. They have contact with ministers of religions and spiritual leaders of diverse convictions. Their contacts with pharmaceutical companies and representatives of medical suppliers are perhaps more indirect and infrequent, but they are no less an essential part of the whole health care industry. As nurses become more flexible in their work, particularly in nurse-led units and practices, nurses have to be more in touch with many more parts of the system.

These trends push nurses to be less inward looking and exclusivist, and, equally, representatives of such agencies need to learn to deal with nurses rather than automatically ask for the doctor. Diversity is opening up fields for us in many directions, widening the vision and giving the possibility for involvement in many more spheres.

It is not only with other professionals and agencies that partnerships have to be forged and developed. The relationships between professionals have to be more in a partnership style. The relationships with clients and patients in particular also need to reflect this. It is increasingly obvious that, for example, clinical trials need to be carried out 'with' people rather than 'on' them; in a similar way, our attitudes to all with whom we work should be in this vein. This not only makes work easier as it creates a better and less stressed atmosphere, but it is also the stance affirming that 'people matter' and is thus a more ethical stance.

In the last chapter, I argued that acting ethically means acting in a visionary, playful, creative way. Here, it should now be clear that such visionary work is also political work because it engages us in areas, fields and work that need our expertise and insights. The model of diagnosis, cure and prognosis is deeply ingrained in the whole of our thinking and acting, not only in medicine. The nursing model has shown that a different approach – one from a starting point of 'people matter' – is again and again more satisfactory and more inclusive. This, too, is an aspect that nurses may have to share with their partners, colleagues and people generally who need more than simply a linear approach to life. The emerging need to forge partnerships is drawing nurses out of their isolation and their undervalued and ignored role. If nurses themselves are not yet making their voice heard, they are being made to make it heard. They are being dragged out of their corner. They should thank the world for it, but they can also lead the world by stepping out and grasping the opportunities. For the sake of their clients and patients, this is indeed ethical work.

Making concerns known

The UKCC *Code of Professional Conduct* (1992a) enjoins on nurses several times that, in the exercise of professional accountability, they must report events and situations that they consider to be contrary to good practice (Clauses 8, 11, 12, 13). 'Whistleblowing' has become a fashionable idea, yet few nurses are in the position to be considered whistleblowers; all of us, however, must make our concerns known, not only because professional practice may be compromised, but also because ethical behaviour is paramount for personal and social well-being.

Whistleblowing came to the fore 'as a symptom of a *general lack of institutional accountability*' (Hunt, 1995, p. 154, original emphasis). An obvious example of this symptom is that nurses have been bound by the UKCC *Code of Professional Conduct* since 1983 (when the first edition of the Code was published), but managers in health care were not similarly bound by any code until 1997. That the symptom even exists:

suggests an organizational culture of intimidation where those with sincere criticisms feel unable to share them. More particularly, it is indicative of a culture which is wilfully self-deceived and wants to believe in the myth of its own goodness. (Pattison, 1997, p. 115)

For the myth to stand, 'an ethos of intimidation and unquestioning obedience' must be maintained. While Pattison argues that this is difficult to impose on public sector workers, Wells (1998, p. 6), speaking for the police, says, 'don't ever doubt the human capacity to obey if backsides, jobs and mortgages are to be kept intact'. The same applies to nursing. Whether perceived or occurring in reality, the message that nurses have picked up is:

> if you are thinking of making a complaint, however legitimate, however appalling the situation about which you wish to complain, then you must expect to be made sick, sacked, financially ruined and at the end of the day your complaint will almost certainly not have been addressed. (Hunt, 1995, p. xvii)

If this is the scenario, why bother?

I may be an optimist, but I believe that few practising nurses are in their jobs only for the money and are unaffected by and unconcerned about anything in their environment or what happens in the profession. Most nurses do bother about, and are bothered by, the many injustices and shortcomings in their working environments. It need not only be open malpractice that concerns nurses. Far more debilitating are constant understaffing, a constant shortage of resources, such as clean linen, not being taken seriously when consulted, or not being consulted at all, and climates in which racism, sexism and ageism are tolerated or even subtly encouraged. All the issues that we take home with us at the end of a day and which stay in our minds and our hearts, causing anger and frustration, are issues that may need to be voiced and aired.

The UKCC document *The Scope of Professional Practice* (1992b) 'increased staff motivation and interest in expanding nurses' role, improved patient care, particularly at night, helped to reduce junior doctors' hours and stress levels and encouraged the development of training programmes' (Jowett, 1997, p. 36) in some trusts. However, Jowett also found that it caused concerns, such as:

- potential pressure, exploitation and abuse
- liability and indemnity
- lack of support from employers
- lack of training opportunities
- public criticism and lack of confidence in nurses
- conflicts with doctors who criticise decisions.

If these issues are actually caused by an official document that should be enhancing for the profession, it is not hard to see that other areas of daily work may potentially cause many more concerns. How and when such concerns are made known depends entirely on the circumstances. What is less conjectural is *that* they should be made known. Most of our efforts and understanding depend on communication, and in this situation, this magic word and aspect is paramount. People matter simply because they are people, and what they mind about and what matters to them matters. Therefore, when someone has a concern, it matters that the concern is voiced and that, with it, the person is listened to and heard. The right to be listened to and heard is a basic human right.

A huge problem with making concerns known is that this inevitably involves other people and exact details. The more detailed we have to be, the more issues become split, and the more blame is sought and applied. Our culture lays great stress on blame and guilt, and on the justice to make it right. This usually means that we hunt for the last detail, the last person who has made a mistake or a wrong decision, and this person is then dismissed or punished. When we are concerned with people more than with blame, we find different values. People work in systems, and when things go wrong, it is not necessarily the people who are at fault but the system. It is less easy to correct a system than it is a single individual, but when a system is 'sick', it is not made better by eliminating one person. Making concerns known is therefore an act of 'healing' the system more than simply curing a disease. A model that starts with 'people matter'' is more applicable in such situations than a model concentrating on diagnosis. Making concerns known – and whistleblowing – are essential aspects of nursing. Dealt with in a way that is based on the principle that people matter, and that mattering matters, they are, above all, ethical acts.

The lack of institutional accountability is an aspect of public life that needs to be addressed urgently and generally. As organisations and institutions are getting bigger through mergers, the less accountable and the more difficult to challenge they are becoming. This also means that it is more necessary that they can be and are challenged. The ethical stance in such organisations may indeed be the political one. This does not mean attacking for the sake of attacking. The Irish politician Edmund Burke (1729-97) is credited with saying, 'It is necessary only for the good man to do nothing for evil to triumph.' I am not implying that organisations are evil. What I am emphasising is that not making concerns known, keeping silent and trying to be 'good' in doing so may not be ethical.

'Proper selfishness'

The term 'proper selfishness' is borrowed from Handy (1997), one of today's management gurus, and, according to Pattison (1997, p. 141), one of the more colourful ones. Pattison considers several such gurus in his book, describing Handy's message as:

> essentially a very simple 'revolutionary' one: the future is going to be increasingly changeable for society and organizations and we are going to have to change with it, making the most of the opportunities that we can provide for ourselves.

I will use here some headings under which Handy (1997, pp. 210–28) considers education, and I will apply them to nursing.

1. 'The discovery of oneself is more important than the discovery of the world'

Handy (p. 210) quotes what Nelson Mandela said in his Inaugural Address:

> Our deepest fear is not that we are inadequate, our deepest fear is that we are powerful beyond measure. We ask ourselves, 'who am I to be brilliant, gorgeous, talented and fabulous?' Actually, who are you not to be? You are a child of God. We are born to manifest the glory of God that is within us. It's not just in some of us, it's in everyone.

In his comment on the passage, Handy (p. 211) says that 'this sentiment, whether put in a religious context or not, should be one of the articles of belief of a school for life and work'. This reflects what I have described in Chapter 1. As nurses, we are aware of our fears, and we can above all empathise with the feelings of the people whom Mandela addressed. The fears of using our considerable powers – positive and negative, light and shadow – are very real in nursing. When we hear our own voice affirmed, we can move mountains. Indeed, we do it every day; too often, we give the credit to others, however, and this is not helpful to them or to us in the long run. Our 'proper selfishness' is part of how we use our political and ethical power. Let us celebrate ourselves.

2. 'Everyone is good at something'

Handy lists many different areas in which we have intelligence: we have factual, numerate, intuitive, athletic, mental, interpersonal, practical and many other kinds of intelligence. In nursing, we have above all relationship intelligence, compassionate intelligence and a huge amount of practical, factual, analytic and preventive intelligence. We know how to be flexible and adapt, and, above all, how to care for people in sickness, vulnerability and illness. Our intelligence ranges over vast areas of life and all ages, giving us insights into the functioning of systems and living that few other professions can claim. When put to the test, most nurses would probably admit to be able to be far more creative than they need to be for their everyday work. If nobody will put us to the test, we need to do it ourselves.

'Political' work is not only standing on rostrums and making speeches. It involves the art of communication, using motivation in an astute way, being prudent and discreet, perhaps knowing when the right moment has arrived for some action. It may even be cunning, in the sense of using stratagems to accomplish a purpose. Political work engages the whole person simply because it uses so many aspects of our intelligence. When we can assert the things at which we are good (rather than bemoan the ones at which we are not), we have perhaps taken the first political step and, in the process, also taken the ethical step because we have asserted that 'people matter'.

3. 'Life is a marathon, not a horse race'

The idea that we have to put ourselves and others to the test at every stage in life is often counterproductive. Many nurses find that they simply cannot keep up with their peers in achieving ever higher educational standards. Achieving good academic grades is very important and shapes future careers, but, when the chips are down, it matters not if someone has a 2:2 or a 2:1; what matters is how the person can face life at a given moment. Higher, further and life-long education are vitally important, but this is not all that there is to nursing.

The idea that life is a journey rather than a destination, a marathon rather than a quick race, is vitally important. It means that all our actions, and not only those that have quick outcomes, are important. Our relationships are important because they influence us. Our words matter because our memories are potent aspects of who we are. Some people are naturally more the 'plodding' type and some more the 'sprinting' type. Both of these are important in the whole scheme of things. Both make important contributions to the web of life; it is just that the contributions are different.

4. 'Knowing "what" is not as important as knowing "where", "how" and "why"'

This aspect of Handy's list is clearly and directly relevant to school education. However, when applied to the idea that political work in nursing is essential, it fits admirably. For any work that is pioneering, making a fresh or different point or involving change, a good deal of 'savvy' is needed. One needs to know one's onions.

Some people have an instinctive knowledge of using people, systems, influence and advertising to the best effect. They may perhaps be the 'naturals' in political work. For other people, making the necessary connections or using networks is not so obvious. The idea of partnerships is therefore very important here because what one person may not know, another may, two heads have always been better than one, and three may be better still.

In political work within nursing it often also helps to know 'who' one knows. Addressing a request to the right person may help to save time and physical and mental energy. Similarly, having access to a person who knows the right person, the friend who has a friend, is important. Even if such people are not available or not known, we should not be deterred. The learning gained in such groundwork is sometimes as important as arriving straight away. Whatever the circumstances, the point is that the 'thing' in itself is not the whole thing, the surrounding elements also matter. We need to consider the 'organic' elements: as a plant needs soil to surround its roots, so an idea needs 'nutrients' of different kinds to grow.

5. 'School should be like work, and vice versa'

Handy is concerned that children are 'not seen as workers, but as the products of... human factories' (p. 220), that is, schools. He wondered what would happen if children were treated as 'the real workers in an enlightened factory of creativity, with the teachers as the consultants and senior managers'. He has an answer: 'accountability and responsibility would then become live concepts, with consequences, because it would be the students, as well as the teachers, who would have to live with [the] consequences' (p. 220). Work would be organised around tasks and in small teams or groups, with competition between groups but co-operation within them. This is essentially what is happening in the health services, but the group or team identity does not often encourage much co-operation.

If school and work were not split into separate concepts, each would benefit from the ideas of the other much more and be involved more with each other. The idea of citizens being involved (Chapter 5) in education, and indeed in every sphere of learning, may become more and more important.

6. 'Life is a journey, which starts at home'

The idea that 'mattering is more given than chosen', explored in Chapter 3, means that, at many times during life, we are confronted with situations that we cannot change but which radically affect our lives. Each of these situations demands a new round of introspection, bringing us 'home' perhaps with a jolt. We have to re-evaluate what we are or who we are to ourselves and others. Some people welcome such jolts, while others find them difficult.

The other side of the metaphor is of course that, in life, we are natural wanderers, discoverers, travellers. It is our natural curiosity that keeps us on the move. At regular intervals, however, we need to reorientate ourselves and look for new challenges and horizons. These points are crucial because they help us to see life from new angles. Some such moments may lead us to think differently or to decide that we really must take some action. They propel us forward on our journey, whatever the journey is. The interplay between travel and rest, expansion and reduction, is not just one of opposites but one of parts of the same whole that is a person.

In terms of ideas concerning political action, it is often at such 'moments of truth' that we are confronted with need and the conviction 'I can do no other'. The journey and the resting times will have contributed to creating the climate in which a conviction is translated into action, or a need has become so strong that we can no longer ignore it. Both situations demand ethical thinking, leading to ethical action, which in this context may be political action.

7. 'Learning is experience understood in tranquillity'

In this part of his chapter, Handy gives his imagination a very good airing. He imagines schools called universities (making school 'respectable'), providing every young person with a mentor from outside the system to be a positive role model and seeing schools as preparing people to 'be responsible for our own destiny, our own definition of success, our own journey of discovery' (p. 228). While this seems to be an exciting way forward, we also have to accept that the reality will never match the ideal; it rarely does. The point of ethical action is precisely here: ethics is about the possible as much as about 'what is'.

In nursing, too, we have to aim for ways and means of being responsible for our own destiny, both personally and professionally. Codes and policies help us, but they can also stifle us. We need to stay involved professionally to achieve this.

We need to aim at defining what success means for us. Is advanced practice the same as expanded practice? What of the nurses who are not in environments where such terms are easily applicable, such as the care of elderly people and of people with learning disabilities? Success in such fields may be measured very differently.

Some people do not like to accept that nursing research, especially when it is qualitative research, is of equal value to scientific and quantitative research. Is it right that two totally different kinds of research have to be measured with the same instruments? Can we not set up different instruments and feel good about being different? If we apply only the known, we can never know what may lie beyond the known. Success is not only of one kind. We may need to find new ways of measuring, comparing and rewarding 'success'. Maybe even a new type of language is necessary for such elements. This is not only academic work, but also political work because the reverberations will be enormous when we dare to challenge the known systems.

In nursing, we are certainly on our own journey of discovery, but we have not yet dared to go very far. We need to open the door of our collective person and step out into that world, telling the world what we discovered while we were inside. That in itself is a political act because the world needs to hear what we have to say.

To balance this section of optimistic ideas, it must be said that 'proper selfishness', like most aspects discussed in this book, has its shadow side. Sometimes the creative 'no' has to be spoken, maybe forcefully. Sometimes proper selfishness needs to be asserted with industrial action, which in itself is also political action. Nurses had long prided themselves that they would not go on strike, and they were able to use this as a bargaining tool for pay settlements in the UK. When the RCN abolished its no-strike rule in 1995, a watershed was reached.

In a whole issue devoted to industrial action, the journal *Nursing Ethics* (1997) featured articles from a world-wide selection of authors, many of whom agonised over the issue of strike action. When nurses strike, they are accused of self-interest, yet nurses say that they are putting patients first. Can the two concepts be squared? Bickley (1997, p. 309) quotes a personal statement in O'Connor (1994):

> I'm on strike because for the last five years my public health system has been whittled away and it has been done by attacking nursing. Effectively we've taken pay cuts for the last three years... It's the first time I've been on strike and I've never felt like this. But I feel justified in taking the action. We had no choice.

This quote sums up many of the really hard problems for nurses: being attacked from outside, being taken for granted, being unable to work effectively because of being restrained by the system, being made to feel guilty for being 'selfish'. Yet when all these come together, a boiling point is reached, and it is not simply one nurse who feels like this but all nurses. The person starts off by speaking for her- or himself and ends speaking for a group. When it matters most, nurses can work together and do have a group identity, even though this is often considered to be lacking.

There are plenty of other ways of taking industrial action: strikes are not the only possibility. Nurses have collected signatures, boycotted dining rooms, not taken holidays, rotated the areas to be targeted and relieved each other on shifts so that they could demonstrate. There are as many possibilities as there are nurses and places of work. The more innovative the action, the more memorable it will be and perhaps the more likely are clients and patients to support it. Indeed, the support and co-operation of users is crucially important.

Industrial action *per se* is political action, but politics is also involved in the manner in which this action is taken. The way in which the action itself is communicated matters, but what matters more is that the message that needs to be given is communicated, that is, said and heard. It has to be unambiguous and focused. When it can be made clear that the real reason for any action is that people matter – clients, patients, nurses, in short all of us – such action will have more chances of getting across and being heard. The political work lies in pushing the ethics out.

Political action

Political action does not have to be spectacular. It should by now
be clear that I consider even small acts of caring to be 'political'
actions. However, it may be useful to point out some possibilities of direct action that may be taken in pursuit of an issue or
principle. The following are not listed in any order of priority:

- It is an ethical and professional duty that our collective and
  individual voice is heard. We owe it to ourselves, our clients,
  patients, colleagues, profession and society that we are not
  overlooked but treated equally. That in itself is a necessary
  ethical and political act
- On occasions, we have to be sure that we say 'no', especially to
  exploitation and misuse. Being treated unfairly and unjustly
  is never acceptable. When clients and patients in our care are
  at risk, we have to use the advocacy role and challenge the
  people concerned. This is not simply an ethical duty, but also
  a political act
- Sometimes a group of people is stronger than an individual;
  groups can be dismissed less easily. Grouping together for
  action is a political act, but it is also a supportive act, and this
  is strengthening the resolve, the bond and the action itself
- Individuals and groups can write letters to relevant people.
  Members of Parliament are often targeted for action. Even if
  no action is taken, at least they have to reply to every letter
  received. If they are made aware of particular incidences,
  they can be very helpful
- Talking with journalists on local papers has often been useful.
  The only thing to be careful of is confidentiality, particularly
  concerning patients
- Lobbying Members of Parliament tends to be effective when a
  group of people are affected. Closing even a few beds in a
  local hospital may be devastating for the community. Protests
  can achieve a great deal. Making the time and action to be
  taken known beforehand to newspapers or journals may
  ensure that the national news media hear about it
- Using organisations such as trade unions and professional
  associations can be very helpful in disputes or disagreements.
  They can give practical and specific support and may take up
  a cause that is brought to them

- When unions and associations seem to lag behind, they may need to be challenged. What are they doing about a particular issue, event or problem? If you do not know the name of a person who could help, telephone the switchboard, ask the operator for the relevant name and then ask to speak to them directly
- Some associations contact their members when particular issues are being discussed in parliaments and other relevant places so that nurses can go along to hearings and sessions, and be supportive. If your association is not imaginative in such ways, ask them why not and what they intend to do about it
- Looking for sponsorship to visit relevant conferences, writing articles in relevant journals and waving banners and placards all help to make particular points and raise consciousness over issues that should concern more people
- Many of these ideas involve much talking in small groups and footwork among colleagues. However, this is necessary for any change to happen. It also helps to formulate ideas and clarify issues, possibly even averting blunders.

The possibilities for political action are as numerous as the reasons themselves. The more imaginatively an issue can be viewed, the more impact it may have. Many of the 'new' ideas for advancing practice clearly come into this area. We should never forget that ideas sometimes also come from the most unexpected sources, and patients sometimes have the best ones yet. After all, the hospice movement grew from the idea of a patient. This clearly shows that listening to ideas and hunches is important because a little time spent 'bending one's ears' may lead to great changes to be enjoyed by millions.

One of the lessons that many people say they learn in tricky situations is that, on their own, they could not have done it. They needed the support of others. Nursing is not known for its care of colleagues. This issue will be addressed in the next chapter. It needs to be said here, however, that if we want to make a political impact, we need to do it together, and this means first of all being supportive of each other. Support, politics and ethics march together.

8

The Ethical is the Supportive

I am writing this only a few days after the funeral of a friend. At least 250 people were present, and most of us knew each other. It was said during the service, and we all knew it for ourselves: Gary had a remarkable gift of making every person feel important. He managed to bring out the best in everybody. One person said that he changed her life in half a minute by just casually asking the right question. Another person admitted that he never knew friendship until Gary came into his life. Many years ago, Gary put me in charge of a working group when I had never done anything like that before. This simple act of trust and addressing the potential rather than only the visible was for me the beginning of a sense of appreciating myself and others differently.

The last chapter made the point that we – all people, and nurses in particular – need to have the right not only to 'voice' concerns, but also to speak generally. The ideas developed so far – that 'people matter' is a basis for nursing to move forward on and that being visionary and politically active is a consequence of this principle – need to be rounded off by seeing them in the context of relationships and supportive action. Only when this is also present can the whole thesis be considered to be ethically valid. One aspect alone is possible in each case but not for holistic work; for that to be possible, we need all aspects to link, support being simply part of the whole. All these elements can only work effectively when they relate to and link in with each other: one is not more important than the other, but each needs to be present for the others to function. By concentrating on support in this chapter, the cycle can be seen to be at work.

The right to free speech is a fundamental human right, but there is more to it than that. We need to talk with each other, respond to each other, express ourselves and communicate our thoughts and feelings. This means that we need to have this right acknowledged by being heard and listened to. Many of us occasionally speak to ourselves, and it is perhaps just as well that, in such moments, nobody hears us. Too many people, however, want to speak and nobody wants to hear them. Too many people also *need* to speak, because they have something important to say, and nobody listens. This sort of talking and 'voicing' is frustrating, demoralising and utterly demeaning. If we have a right to free speech and to express ourselves, we have the equal right to be heard. The trouble is that communicating takes time, and this is what many of us no longer have. Perhaps the most important thing that we can give to someone is our time. It need not be a long time, but it needs to be quality time.

Nurses' supportive work

Every definition of what nurses do or nursing is points to support. Nurses support clients and patients in their illness, with the aim of achieving either better health or a peaceful death, or of finding ways and means of coping with what is given. All nursing care is supportive care: supporting the person with the illness at the time of needing to adjust to new and sometimes frightening circumstances. In this, then, we have the thesis that I have used throughout this book: people matter, mattering matters, and mattering is more given than chosen.

In UK nursing, the most quoted lines must surely be the 'stem' sentence in the UKCC (1992a) *Code of Professional Conduct*:

> As a registered nurse, midwife or health visitor, you are personally accountable for your practice and, in the exercise of your professional accountability must...

Here, put in words of duty, the supportive role of nurses is seen as an ethical imperative. If we do not conform to these standards, we are liable to be punished. Indeed, in the year ended 31 March 1998, the UKCC removed 84 people from the register for reasons of:

physical or verbal abuse of patients and clients (31% of removals), failure to attend to basic needs (13%), unsafe clinical practice and patient abuse (both 7%). (UKCC, 1998b)

If these examples show what unprofessional practice is, they also show what 'un-supportive' care is.

The essential role of nurses is to support other people in their need: to nourish, nurture, protect and promote emotional growth (Chapter 4). It is to stand by others in their need and at their most vulnerable times and occasions. These actions are more often seen as kindness and altruism than as an ethical duty. It may be understandable that they are an ethical duty for doctors, who, after all, get well paid for this work. However, nurses do the same acts and get paid much less for them. It may be said that nurses' hours are more regulated than those of physicians, but nurses regularly work through their meal breaks and do unpaid overtime, saving the NHS millions of pounds (Buchan, 1991). Indirectly therefore nurses are also supporting the NHS as an organisation.

Nurses not only work hard out of altruism and do overtime out of kindness: they do it because there is satisfaction in what they do; they feel affirmed and recognised. Subjectively, these are good reasons for doing the kind of work that nurses do, but this is only one aspect of work. We cannot gain all our income and respectability by making our feelings work for us. The objective reasons for going into nursing and staying there have to do with a belief in humanity at a much wider level than that of the individual, and with a reasoning for alleviating humanity's sufferings that is wider than the task at hand. Nursing is a commitment to life altogether and an engagement with the world that is wider and bigger than the individual nurse. The UKCC Code asks us to act professionally and to 'serve the interests of society'. If the word 'serve' were replaced with 'engage with' society, the emphasis would be entirely different, considering nursing a 'political' force to reckon with.

The code of ethics for nurses in Australia (Australian Nursing Council, 1993) says, under Value statement 6 ('Nurses value the promotion of an ecological, social and economic environment which supports and sustains heath and well-being'):

Nursing includes involvement in the detection of ill effects of the environment on the health of persons, the ill effects of human activities on the natural environment, and assisting communities on their actions on environmental health problems aimed at minimizing these effects.

In this code, nurses are exhorted to think in wider terms and see nursing within a wider setting, thus effectively supporting the smooth running of society as a whole. If we consider that 'people matter', this applies to all spheres of life.

> Nurses and nursing do a vital job of supporting not only individuals, but also institutions and systems so that life can be lived as freely, effectively and satisfyingly as possible. As in natural ecosystems, if one layer is removed, the whole system collapses; thus, if nursing as a profession were to disappear, major realignments would be necessary. Rather than contemplating such a scenario, nursing must be concerned with the effective running and interaction of all the systems. In this way, not only is nursing vital, but also its supportive role is an ethical one.

Just as nursing therefore has to support the beneficent structures, it has a duty to question the maleficent ones. Ethical behaviour demands vigilance and a constant attunement to society as a whole, one's environment and oneself. This does not mean spying or snooping but listening and hearing what is being said and done. Perhaps the response might most often actually be recognition and a thank you, as this is perhaps the most supportive thing that we can do. When this is not possible, we should not tolerate situations that are undermining good behaviour or demeaning persons.

The supportive work of nurses is as wide as society and as particular as the individual. It is the essential 'midwife' role of empowering people and organisations to be able to act in accordance with their conscience, beliefs and values, and to challenge situations and behaviours that militate against this. This work clearly has to be done in an informed manner, and therefore life-long education – both personally and professionally –

is not simply a prescription but an ethical way of being and seeing. Sofaer (1994, p. 173) wondered whether, as nurses, we are our 'brothers' keepers', that is, whether we have a moral obligation to achieve a better life on the planet. She sees this role mainly in the way in which nurses intervene in disasters and situations where human rights are violated. She believes that nurses have traditionally picked up the pieces from inhuman actions and ecological disasters. In this role, nurses have supported people admirably. Sofaer's (1994, p. 177) conclusion, however, is that the concern of nurses for the sick and dying:

> *could* and *should* be harnessed further as a concern for the welfare of the human race. We do not only have a right to intervene, we are obliged to do so. If we do not act as individuals and as professional carers and educators, who will? When we witness and recognise such situations, we have a moral obligation to act as nurses and as human beings. We are our 'brothers' keepers'.

A part of the challenge of nursing will always be the question 'Who will do it?' or 'Who will go there?', and the ethical response is 'I will.' Nursing is a kind of anticipating the question 'Will you help me?' from a sick or helpless person; it is anticipating a loss of human dignity by preventing the situation occurring. The supportive role therefore stretches beyond the individual pain or misery to the wider concern.

Not only do nurses have to acknowledge that they have this role of supporting and nurturing, but they also have to have it acknowledged by other professionals. We cannot give what we have not got; that is, we cannot support others if we are not supported. That must surely be the first ethical stance to take and give.

The supportive role of management

When we say that 'nurses care', we are essentially saying that nurses care for other people, and not themselves. When we make an 'ethic of care' the starting point for nursing, we lose the argument because all health workers 'care'. However, when we consider that 'people matter' and that 'mattering matters', we start from a different angle altogether, because 'people' means everybody, including nurses (that is, ourselves), managers, politicians and clients. Rather than stressing one aspect of nurses' work, the stress is on the inclusive nature of being human.

In order to make it explicit, I believe many nurses have gone into management, hoping in that way to change the climate and make it more 'kind' and supportive. As discussed in the last chapter, this does not, however, seem to work because managers do not have enough power to change a climate and thus leave before they can make their ideals reality. Some form of political action might get them further because they could aim deeper and more radically than the managerial layer of responsibility.

For years, it seemed that the word 'support' was somehow not quite acceptable or was applicable only to those poor souls who could not stand the heat. The NHS in particular seems to have learned a lesson in the past few years. Once business generally began to make it clear that its workforce was its most valuable asset, the trickle-down effect was inevitable. It takes a while, however, to turn a big ship like the NHS round to head off in another direction, although thankfully, this is now happening (Secretary of State for Health, 1997).

When nurses are not able to practise professionally as they are intending or hoping, they feel angry, guilty (Fairbairn and Mead, 1990, p. 11) and powerless. Stoter (1995, p. 146) claims that:

> when stress is allowed to build up unchecked, the balance [between healthy and unhealthy stress] is disturbed, the point of creativity is passed and there is a negative response which can have all kinds of undesirable effects.

Support for staff is therefore not only a restorative function, but also a necessity to keep the workforce physically and mentally healthy and functioning. Staff support may be a tool of enlightened self-interest, but it is also more than that: it is an ethical imperative if we work from the premise that 'people matter'. If regulators of the profession and managers of organisations ask nurses (and other care staff) to support patients and clients, they need to support the staff. Those (politicians and managers) who ask others (nurses) to do a job that is the politicians' and managers' ultimate responsibility (that is, to care for the sick in society) need to ensure that those delegated to do the work can do it, both physically and emotionally. The managers' responsibility to their own managers and their electorate demands that they take their responsibility towards their workforce seriously. The privileges that they enjoy as part of their job demands that they take their own responsibilities seriously.

Managers may of course argue that they have not been given the resources to care for their staff. They neither have the money to employ counsellors and therapists of different categories, nor the leeway to give staff the time to attend such sessions or have more time free for leisure or other forms of self-development. The spiral of 'not enough' becomes ever deeper and tighter, yet the cost involved in absenteeism and sickness among staff who are stressed and burned out vastly exceeds that of supplying support. The National Association for Staff Support (1992a, p. 5) figures speak for themselves, particularly when considering their date of publication:

> Sickness and absenteeism alone costs business approximately £5bn per year. (Confederation of British Industry, 1987)

> One million people are missing from offices or factories every day which costs British industry £6 billion per year. Many of those missing million will be doing so either to sort out personal problems or because they are too depressed to work. (Anderson, 1991)

> Losing and replacing experienced nurses is costing the NHS up to £24 million every year... The RCN survey shows each nurse leaver costs the health service an average £3,000. It puts the annual turnover at an average of 25%, equal to 80,000 nurses, and reveals savings as high as £6.4 million could be made by cutting the rate to 15% nationally. (RCN, 1991)

In 1998, the Nuffield Trust (Williams *et al.*, 1998) published the findings of the 'most extensive survey of research ever undertaken into the health of the NHS workforce' and found 'worrying' trends, such as 'a considerably higher incidence of ill health in the NHS workforce than in other occupations'. Their evidence concerning nurses is just as grim:

High levels of psychological disturbance, ranging from emotional exhaustion to suicide, exist in 29% to 48% of nurses. The level of psychological disturbance is significantly higher in nurses than in equivalent professional groups in the general population. Emotional exhaustion predicts sickness absence and has doubled in community nurses between 1991 and 1995.

Most nurses experience back pain at some time which is associated with high absenteeism, staff turnover and ill health retirement. This problem has increased by almost 40% from 1983 to 1995. (p. 19)

The Report's (Williams *et al.*, 1998, p. 24) own figures relate to numbers nearer to its date of publication:

Sickness absence rates of 5% or more are costing the NHS over £700 million a year. ...British industry averages around 3.7% sickness absence. If the NHS could cut down sickness by only one percentage point, or about two and a half days per staff member per year, it could save itself over £140 million a year or the equivalent of 1% of pay.

The sources of ill health among nurses are listed as:

high workload, workload pressures and their effect on personal lives, staff shortages, unpredictable staffing and scheduling and not enough time to provide emotional support to patients. Poor management style including impatience, defensiveness, unsupportive leadership, lack of feedback and clarity and giving insufficient control. Distress in student nurses caused by low involvement in decision-making and use of skills and low social support at work. (p. 21)

When this list is read with 'people matter' in mind, there remain very few points not directly related to an infringement of its principles. In other words, believing and maintaining that 'people matter' is basic to human interaction and relationships. In this light, it can also be seen that the dictum 'people matter' is indeed the basic ethical stance for contact with people. When we say that 'people matter', we say it of others and of ourselves.

- If a nurse says that people matter, this nurse affirms her or his care of patients and clients.
- If a manager says that people matter, this manager affirms her or his care of the people he or she manages.

- If a director or executive says that people matter, this person affirms that the people he or she directs or manages matter.
- What goes up in the hierarchy also comes down in the hierarchy, and in this way everybody says of themselves and of others that they matter. This must be the basic pledge of any person in any charge of other persons.

The supportive role of management is therefore a duty to support under the principle that 'people matter'.

There will always be stress and problems, but many of the stressors listed above need not exist, at least not permanently. Many of the reasons for stress exist because of bad communication or simply a disregard for or inattention to the fact that people matter. When we take each other for granted or treat each other as figures, numbers or simply resources, we can fall into the trap of losing sight of 'people matter'. One such trap is indeed the department now generally known as 'human resources'. While this may be an improvement on the term 'personnel' because at least the human side is acknowledged, people are more than just a resource. The language used to describe something or someone in itself influences the atmosphere and culture of any organisation.

I will describe below some of the measures and actions that are particularly supportive to staff in health care. It is very often not the extraordinary actions or statements that count but the personal touch. It is this which people will remember for good or ill. Even a small hurt can go very deeply. Being overlooked or made to feel unimportant may seem a small item, but it is that which shows whether or not people matter. Making someone 'feel like a person, you know, not a number' (Morrison and Burnard, 1997, p. 89) counts. If not, what will be remembered will be, 'the thing that really hurt was [that] nobody said: "Please don't go"' (Carlisle, 1997, p. 27) when cutbacks had to be made. It is often not *what* is done so much as *how* it is done which counts in relationships.

That management has a clear responsibility to support staff is not, or at least is no longer, in question. Whether it does it is another question. The National Association for Staff Support and other bodies have worked diligently to make nurses aware of their need and right to support, and management of their duties. A clause in *A Charter for Staff Support* (National Association for Staff Support, 1992b, p. 5) makes the point that:

> Staff are entitled to have access to immediate debriefing facilities following any traumatic situation and to have such facilities available as part of a normal daily service.

The subsequent clause states that:

> Managers at all levels need to be educated about counselling skills and to be sensitive to staff needs so they can ensure that the appropriate support is available.

Many of the supportive measures are neither expensive nor difficult to access. They may take a little personal endeavour, imagination and empathy. 'Do unto others as you would be done by' is not simply a quaint piece of good advice; it is actually a powerful and global means of maintaining justice.

Clinical supervision

I am singling out clinical supervision as a form of support that is unique. The personal and intimate contact with someone who is concerned entirely with that person's well-being is far more decisive and supportive than any other form of support possible in the workplace. The other possibilities of supervision used in nursing, such as mentorship and preceptorship, are well established and are normally used in situations of training and learning. They are therefore different from clinical supervision, which is used for qualified staff who, to all intents and purposes, do not need practice in skills and guidance with tasks.

The main question that Fowler (1996, p. 384) asks is 'what is the aim of clinical supervision?' He goes on to list several different frameworks, each having merit when viewed from that angle. De Raeve (1998, p. 489) believes that the aim of clinical supervision is:

essentially to enable nurses to work with moral integrity in their role and... supervisors need, therefore, to be people with a reasonable degree of integrity themselves.

She bases this on the fact that:

in caring for sick, ill, dependent, demanding, needy, dying, grateful and ungrateful people, nurses are exposed to sometimes physical and frequently psychological threats to their integrity which render it difficult to sustain the moral focus of nursing and preserve the capacity to nurse with integrity.

Her argument is therefore that:

clinical supervision, when done well by people adequately trained and with adequate support for themselves, provides a forum for the preservation or restoration of integrity in nursing.

De Raeve mentions different aspects of integrity: bodily, spiritual, psychological and moral. It is this latter which she sees as having to do with our adherence to moral values and therefore as being tied to our sense of dignity and self-respect. This aspect too is stressed in the thesis that 'people matter'.

If clinical supervision is to be effective and acceptable, it has also to be regulated. Dimond (1998b, p. 395) believes that the UKCC needs to give a clear lead on the subject. This is related to Fowler's (1996, p. 382) point that:

many of us have experience of the elements that make up clinical supervision, but we often lack experience and confidence in putting them all together and taking on the formal role of clinical supervisor. In essence, many of us are not sure what to do after we sat [sic] down with our supervisee and said 'hello'.

What accountability is there in the role? What are the time and money factors involved? Do patients have the right of access to the record of supervision? Indeed, what records are kept and by whom? Who writes them? If patients and clients are discussed, what are the issues concerning confidentiality? (Cain, 1997, pp. 465–71). What are the actual and perceived problems with setting up clinical supervision? (Bishop, 1998, p. 51). When such issues and topics are clarified, such supervision must surely be seen as an important tool of support and integrity.

Fowler (1996, p. 382) cites Proctor's (undated) framework in which she identifies three areas of supervision: formative, normative and restorative. However, the interpretation that Fowler puts on these aspects is very narrow.

The formative aspect of clinical supervision needs to relate directly to practice, Lowry (1998, p. 553) mentioning in particular its role 'to identify solutions to problems, improve practice and increase understanding of professional issues'. Peer evaluation and peer review are well established practices in all professional life, but, for many nurses, the supervision they have been used to is that from a teacher or superior while they were students. The idea therefore that a peer and someone equal in the hierarchical ladder can be and is a supervisor needs some adjustment in thinking and relating, for both supervisor and supervisee. This may, however, be a most important learning experience on the way to accepting all people as equal. If we say that 'people matter', this means that all people matter equally. While in theory there is no problem in affirming this, in practice we all know that we make distinctions, and, as professionals, we are peculiarly prone to treating our clients as less understanding or knowledgeable. The formative elements of clinical supervision may specifically refer to practice and actual problems encountered with clients and patients, but we must not forget that these problems often arise because of our own mind-set and attitude. Testing these out against a peer can therefore be a lesson in itself. The potential problem and challenge is that the same person is likely to be both supervised and a supervisor for others. It therefore takes integrity to be honest in both roles.

The normative aspect of supervision refers to the part that clinical supervision plays in maintaining the professional in his or her integrity: physical, in that the person's health is noted; spiritual, in that the two people are able to discuss matters of meaning and importance, especially when challenged by a traumatic experience; psychological, in that any stress is noted, voiced and heard; and moral, in that issues of conscience, justice and dignity can be aired and debated. Undoubtedly, the tension caused by the dual role of each person also has to be considered.

The restorative aspect, according to Fowler (1996, p. 383), concerns the 'responsibility for ensuring the supervisee is adequately refreshed and supported'. This statement seems to miss some of the point of this important element. Minor breaches of confidentiality, not reporting drug errors for fear of being dealt with too harshly (Wilson, 1998) or having taken a personal risk in the A & E department with a person carrying a weapon because the person was known to the nurse – such incidences may be ideally considered in clinical supervision and there dealt with satisfactorily, restoring the nurse in question to the integrity needed to carry on the work. Too often when such incidences occur, they are blown out of proportion, with devastating consequences, helping nobody and possibly adding to an atmosphere of fear and mistrust, deviousness and dishonesty. On the other hand, when such problems cannot be aired, nurses carry the sentiments with them, possibly for years, often leaving guilt and self-doubt behind. This is not only emotionally costly, but may also ruin a career in nursing (Anonymous, 1998b, p. 19).

It must be clear from this that agreements must be established on what supervision is, what it aims to do and what its legal status is. If a supervisor can deal with such incidences, she or he needs to have this role and status acknowledged. The last aspect discussed may in fact lead to further action and possibly disciplinary proceedings, so the supervisor needs to know clearly what limits are imposed on the role and what privileges are granted. Cutliffe *et al.* (1998, pp. 920–3) consider that guidelines are necessary in clinical supervision as some practice may cause ethical dilemmas. There are likely to be few such situations, but they need to be anticipated and minimised, otherwise harm may be caused.

Clinical supervision is only one possibility – but a strong one – for changing the climate of an organisation to a supportive one:

> Having an open, honest and blame-free organisation which is open to improving processes and systems of care is a big step towards having staff who are committed to quality and getting things right. (Wilson, 1998, p. 670)

This may be a wish, but it is certainly one to strive for. If clinical supervision is to enable nurses to work with integrity, 'clinical supervision offers a radical challenge to nursing's existing culture. If nurses are interested in the survival of the profession, it is perhaps a challenge that has to be grasped' (de Raeve, 1998, p. 495).

Over the years, many authors have used Campbell's (1984, p. 49) ideas of 'skilled companionship' as an important concept for taking nursing forward, but it has never quite caught on. Maybe in calling it clinical supervision the notion has finally been seen for what it is: the force for change that can liberate nursing because it is seen no longer as something that happens only between nurses and patients, but as something that applies to nurses themselves. When nurses learn to be skilled companions to each other, they will then have a much greater sense of self-worth and will be much more empowered to hear their own voice – by listening to each other – and making their voice heard.

Supportive action

A cartoon in *New Internationalist* (1998, p. 5) shows a woman in her pyjamas opening the front door to her husband, giving a glimpse of the moon in the dark sky while a clock on the wall stands at nearly midnight. Sweat is pouring off the husband's head while he staggers through the door, saying 'I loved and supported EVERYONE I met today.' A bubble over the cat, cosy in her basket, says: 'IMPORTANT POINT: Remember to love and support YOURSELF too.' Cats are known for their innate sense of getting what they need. One might wish that the human race – or at least that part of it which is in the caring professions – might at times copy the feline population a little more.

The researchers working on the Nuffield Trust report (Williams *et al.*, 1998, p. 23) identified a number of specific interventions that were considered to be 'methodologically acceptable':

Type of support	*Extent of success*
Training skills to mobilise work-based support and to participate in problem solving and decision making	Improvement in mental health, particularly for those intending to leave
Psychologist provided support, advice and feedback	Reduced stress hormone levels
Communication skills training	Reduced staff resignations, sick leave, assaults and the cost of each of these
Interpersonal awareness training	Reduced emotional exhaustion and depression
Organisational stress management programme	Reduced medical malpractice claims and medication errors
Exercise	Improved well being and reduced complaints of muscle pains particularly for those who are generally inactive
Ergonomic intervention and skills training to prevent and manage musculo-skeletal problems	Cost effective reduction in injuries and absenteeism
Organisational intervention to manage return to work after ill health	Reduced sickness absence with considerable financial savings.

These measures cover the whole of the workforce in the NHS. When considering nurses in particular, certain areas of supportive action need especially to be highlighted. Using here de Raeve's (1998, p. 486) categories of integrity (above) and the services listed by National Association for Staff Support (1992b) in the Charter as existing already and available, a fairly composite picture emerges.

Support for physical integrity

Of the interventions mentioned by the Nuffield Trust report (Williams *et al.*, 1998, p. 23), several areas directly concern physical health and fitness. Nurses generally have had much training in lifting and handling patients, and more suitable equipment constantly comes onto the market. As all nurses know, it is not the planned lifting and moving that is difficult but the unplanned and unexpected movements that have to be made, which catch nurses out and cause the real damage.

Physical fitness alone, however, does not yet cause physical integrity. General health and well-being have to be ensured by both individuals and employers. In the Green Paper *Our Healthier Nation; A Contract for Health,* the Secretary of State for Health (1998) outlines targets and aims for improving the health of the population as a whole. In advocating how work-places can be considered healthy, the following are mentioned as being applicable to employers:

Have excellent standards of health and safety management.

Take measures to reduce stress at work.

Try to create flexible working arrangements that are compatible with employees' home lives and provide childcare facilities.

Ensure a smoke free working environment.

Contribute to and implement the Health and Safety Commission's forthcoming consultation paper on a ten-year strategy for occupational health.

Make healthy choices easy for staff, eg provision for cyclists, healthy canteens. (p. 44)

This list does not contain anything new or startling. What is perhaps more needed than anything in all these areas is for the ideas to be put into practice and people to make use of them. Rather than seeing these recommendations as yet another chore for yet another committee, little more than a bit of imagination and willingness may be needed to correct the situation. In partic-ular, occupational health services are often the cinderella service in health care settings yet could be the place and department that makes all the difference to staff well-being. The support that they can give is vital in most aspects, and sometimes even an aspirin and a chat – the vital 'tea and sympathy' – can be of immense help in keeping one's head. So that support can be given and accepted, staff need to be aware of what services are available, occupational health staff need to be known and the service should preferably be situated somewhere easily accessible.

Support for spiritual integrity

Chaplaincy services fulfil a function that can never be under-estimated in an institution, especially a hospital. The meeting together of suffering and pain, hope and disillusion, fear and loving care can create among staff an atmosphere of indifference as a means of coping and among patients a sense of infantile dependence. The role that chaplains and pastoral care workers of various denominations and faiths play varies greatly depending on their personality and the welcome they get from senior staff, but they need to be versed in more than religious ritual to be able to relate to people in all these states and stages.

The spiritual needs of people are not only fulfilled by religious leaders. Hospital chapels and sanctuaries can be welcoming places, but they can also be off-putting to people and be perceived as being too much tied to a particular expression of spirituality. In times of need, people often do not find what would support them most. To have a wide range of services and agencies available is imperative in any kind of support giving (Stoter, 1995).

Generally speaking, people now have become more at ease with talking about spiritual needs and having these fulfilled in unusual ways. Some people find re-creation and spiritual refreshment and support in walking, dancing or other physical activity. Other people need quiet and are replenished when meditating or praying. Still others find fulfilment in the creative arts. A mundane job, such as cooking, can turn into a spiritual act, and, conversely, praying can be the inspiration for some action that might have been dreaded. The important thing about spiritual support is not the label we give to it but that we are aware of what is happening. If it helps to balance us, and to be persons of integrity again, it will have been supportive, whatever 'it' was.

Albrecht (1982, p. 10) quotes Selye (1976), the great writer on stress, as saying that the need 'for contemplation of something infinitely greater' is one way of diffusing daily frustrations. Albrecht himself, writing about staff nurses, advocates prayer as helping 'individual nurses gain a deeper perspective of themselves and their role as care givers'.

> The need for spiritual support often goes very deep and
> just as often is unacknowledged and unfulfilled. When we
> can and do pay attention to the person, the individual,
> including ourselves, we may quickly get to the point at
> which we realise that 'mattering matters'. What we care
> about is often the very thing that we deny caring about.
> By allowing ourselves to believe that we matter, we give
> ourselves the possibility to get in touch with what matters
> and what we mind about.

One of the means of support to which increasing numbers
of people are turning is spiritual direction or guidance. This
has many aspects similar to those of clinical supervision in that
it is a one-to-one activity. The 'director' (some people prefer
the title 'soul friend') is often a member of the clergy or someone
specially trained. Since the director tends to be seen as an
expert, it may foster a teacher–pupil relationship. However,
Laishley (1998, p. 116) makes the important point that:

> there may be – in most cases it is presumed – an inequality of
> individual experience, but the personal equality giving rise to accep-
> tance, respect and openness is basic. The process seems to me to
> be a shared search. The more familiar activity of teaching offers
> analogies: there may be an element of instruction of one by another
> but it would be a mistake to think of teaching as the transfer of
> knowledge possessed by one to another more ignorant than oneself:
> it is, rather, a matter of the facilitating of learning. Here horizons
> are being pushed back for both participants, and familiar patterns
> of understanding revised.

Like clinical supervision, spiritual guidance tends to be a long-
term relationship. Organisations may not see it as their duty
specifically to supply spiritual guides, but they have them in
their chaplains already, and counsellors and many other people
act as guides and soul friends to others. If it helps people to
be more human and whole beings, surely it should be available. Spiritual dereliction can lead to sickness just as surely as
physical unfitness can, so anything that avoids it must be considered as a legitimate source of support. At least one health
authority in England supports nurses who go on one-day
retreats by paying their fees for them.

Support for psychological integrity

Nurses have used many of the well-known practices of psychological support for years. Counselling skills are part of the nurses' daily repertoire of caring, but they have not been used in the same measure to care for nurses. The mismatch in what is required of nurses and what is required of managers is a clear injustice and may be one of the reasons for dissatisfaction. Lack of staff support, variously expressed, is noted by Wheeler (1998, pp. 40–3) in his review of several major studies concerning stress in nurses.

Before counselling skills can be used by anybody, there has to be a good deal of self-awareness, and interpersonal skills need to be learned and fostered. Courses need to be held for and attended by staff. One of the 'problems' with such skills is that if managers consider so-and-so to be in need of learning such skills, that person is not going to learn them by being told to. It needs inner readiness, and, when that is present, a good deal of awareness is there already. Courses in interpersonal skills and conflict management have to be well run by experienced people and in a creative way, otherwise staff will not be tempted onto them. There should also be follow-up possibilities as such courses can uncover major psychological problems. For professionals dealing with people all the time, the need to learn such skills is imperative and should be encouraged in such a way that the person recognises the need her- or himself.

Attending courses of many kinds is not only professionally stimulating, but also enhances the person's self-esteem. Going on some course may be a cathartic experience and help to determine someone's career. Being asked to attend a course may show that the person is valued. It may be that an appraisal has highlighted a particular need and having this honoured is important.

Job advertisements tend to make claims to the effect that an employer fosters further study and applicants take this seriously. When it then turns out that the employer only means in-house-run courses that do not have official status, new recruits can feel bitterly let down and deceived. Openness and honesty in dealing with staff are fundamental issues in maintaining the staff's psychological health. If staff see that management will do everything to save only its own skin, they too may need to employ the same tactics, thus undermining morale. While we may consider this stance to be cheating, it is also infringing basic ethical principles of justice, truth, individual freedom and beneficence, and is not respecting the principle that people matter.

Support groups and various schemes of having time out are very important if staff are to feel and be valued. Such groups and schemes are endlessly variable and flexible, and perhaps need to be. The danger, when they change, is that staff may be forgotten or overlooked. Nevertheless, such arrangements are sometimes valid only for a time and have to die before they can be started again in an other form. Despite the fact that support is vital, it is not necessarily automatic, and there is as much responsibility placed on those who need it to acquire it as there is on those who provide it to ensure that it is given (Thomas, 1995, pp. 36–9).

Psychological support stresses above all the aspect of the mind, feelings, memory, values, meaning and relating to people and surroundings. When any of these aspects suffer, the whole person suffers. We are all aware of the influence of the mind on the cause and course of disease – and vice versa. If we want to stay psychologically fit, we have to satisfy many needs. We can say that, as nurses, we owe it to our clients and patients to be as healthy as possible in order to care for them adequately. If this means attending a course of study, going on holiday, tending a garden or having enough time for family and friends, these should not be neglected, and employers have to acknowledge this. Indeed, one of the Nuffield Trust report's (Williams *et al.*, 1998, p. 27) recommendations for nurses is to 'introduce family-friendly policies, e.g. career-breaks and support [for] personal development'. It is impossible to separate the various aspects of integrity – indeed, the meaning of integrity is wholeness – but to clarify various aspects can help. Psychological support fosters psychological integrity as part of the one complete integrity.

Many of the support elements that foster psychological integrity are essentially available in organisations, but they are underused and perhaps also not well publicised. If nurses

(and all health care workers) are not to be damaged by
their work and use inappropriate coping strategies, such
as substance misuse, mental illness or even suicide
(Farrington, 1997, p. 44), the onus is on the organisation
to reverse the trends and change the climate to one in
which staff are content and like to work.

Support for moral integrity

Ethics has not always figured highly in nurses' work. A generally increasing demand for clarity and accountability has pushed
the need for ethical thinking and behaviour into the open, not
least because of the media's uncovering of some very unethical behaviour in high places. Nurses are now often well versed
in ethical theories and principles, but they need to be so also
in practice. If we are to argue that supporting their staff is an
ethical duty for employers, we have to have a basis for doing
so. However, much more than this, the need to maintain our
moral integrity and that of our clients, patients, colleagues and
friends has to be based on sound values and beliefs. As professionals, we rightly demand to be involved in decision making
at all levels of our work. This inevitably involves us in making
choices that can sometimes test our integrity. Knowing about
ethical principles and reasoning may not make the choices easier
but may cause us fewer mental problems. I would contend therefore that all nurses need to have some basic knowledge of
ethics and philosophy for their own psychological and moral
well-being.

The use of reflective practice is now well established in
nursing practice, although it may not necessarily include ethical
reflection. Durgahee (1997, p. 140) found that using student
nurses' personal diaries in group settings helped them to:

> question and challenge their established practices, convictions, basic
> beliefs and attitudes, and 'moved them on' as maturing practi-
> tioners and people.

Although students found this sometimes a taxing exercise because they were initially more interested in acquiring facts, Durgahee (1997, pp. 140–1) cites the following remarks made by students, which show that they benefited from the exercise:

> The reflective group helped me to question my values, philosophy and approach to nursing decisions.
>
> Being aware of my beliefs, actions and my practice are crucial in ethical decision-making.
>
> I have learned to reason and think clearly.
>
> Patients must be seen as real people not just patients. Patients need to see nurses as people... not mere nurses doing their job.

Perhaps one of the most helpful supportive aspects of moral integrity is to challenge and question practitioners as people. It is not so much their actions that need to be questioned as their motives, habits, thinking, attitudes, values and beliefs. This should not be an aggressive interrogation as this would be destructive of the person. A challenging questioning, possibly in a group setting, may achieve much more and be more effective. For this to happen, trust and honesty are necessary bases. Thus we are into ethics.

In the classes of postregistration students that I have been teaching for some years, I am constantly surprised how little these nurses connect their daily activities with ethical thinking and acting. They do not see that the way in which they say 'good morning' to colleagues and clients is an ethical act: in the way they behave as if 'people matter', or because the way they are treated by managers may be against basic human rights – if they are not heard, or are threatened if they make concerns known. Johnstone (1998, p. 43) argues that the 'nursing ethics literature has not always reflected the reality of nurses' daily problems', among which she mentions:

> nurses' rights and interests despite the fact that nurses are at disproportionate risk compared with other health workers of being exploited, abused, injured and even killed.

These are the obvious areas that can be found in the media headlines. The more subtle 'daily problems' are largely known only to nurses: all the aspects that have been mentioned in earlier chapters, such as being overlooked, ignored, not involved in decision making – in short, those aspects making up the inequality with other health professionals. While all this may be explained in terms of sociology, for nurses it is also experienced in terms of morality. If we want to get our voice heard, I believe that we have to say this now in terms of ethics and morality. This is the language that is understood today.

> The principle that 'people matter' goes to the heart of all ethical and moral action. As nurses, we have been acting ethically and morally in this light ever since people called themselves nurses. If any support for moral integrity can be given, it is the support to have 'people matter' also applied to us from every quarter. 'Nurses matter' because 'people matter' for ourselves, patients, colleagues, clients and users, employers, regulators, governments and society.

Perhaps one of the first things that we, as nurses, need to do in this scenario is to affirm our voice. It is because the daily, seemingly small gestures and attitudes are of fundamental concern that we have a voice. When we affirm this voice and make it heard – in ethical and moral terms – we also need to make sure that we are being heard. Not being heard is also an infringement of 'people matter'. The outcome of this, I believe, will be a supportive leadership within nursing and of nursing within society. Among the 'everyday' practical ethical issues that Johnstone (1998, p. 43) mentions as being relevant to nursing are:

> the need to advance a genuinely nursing perspective on common mainstream bioethical issues; and the otherwise neglected broader social justice issues associated with promoting the wellbeing and significant moral interests of marginalized groups.

Nurses need to be deeply involved in these issues if nursing as a profession is to remain ethical. Conversely, nurses need to be supported to maintain their moral integrity.

Rowden (1998, p. 24) is noted for his outspoken ways and frank language. At a ward leaders' conference, he said that leaders in nursing are everywhere in hospitals, on executive boards and in universities, but often:

> those who claim leadership of nursing cling to their own outdated views and fail to spot new leaders. The fatal flaw of old-style nursing hierarchies is their ungenerous spirit. They are based on a culture of insecurity, based on over-reliance on patronage, of control, not of empowerment.
>
> There are thousands of nurses honing and using their leadership skills up and down the land but, because of our over-reliance on a control-freak mentality, sustained by rigid notions of hierarchy, we often fail to recognise what leadership is about. Good leadership creates a culture where diversity and dissent are valued, structures are open, ideas and talent can fly and where people empower others.
>
> As we approach the millennium, nursing must have the confidence to escape the treacle of our history.
>
> Look to the leader inside yourself.

Employers cannot say that they will support their employees' physical and mental health but that the spiritual and moral health is beyond them. Supporting people is equivalent to empowering them. If professionals are to be empowered (which they must be, otherwise they are not professionals), they have to be supported physically, spiritually, psychologically and morally. Only then can nurses act with integrity and vision, and challenge systems that do harm, or at least no good. To act ethically is always to be concerned for others as well as for ourselves, and many a time this is also political action. When we say that people matter, we mean everybody. This principle is so powerful because it is inclusive, giving us the insights and the argument to ensure that support is seen as an ethical imperative. Holistic care – given and received – is only possible when all these elements are present and interact.

9

Nurses as Moral Artists

The idea of nursing as a moral art has been mentioned before (Tschudin, 1997, p. 64). Churchill (1994, p. 328) puts it pictorially when he writes that ethical:

> principles are like paintbrushes in the hands of moral artists; the artist should use them to portray the moral landscape and set the contours of our choices, altering the world we see and in which we will act.

I am using the term 'artist' in a very loose way in this chapter. By artists, I obviously mean people who paint, sculpt and write poetry, dance and make music, but I also mean people who cook a lovely meal, create a relaxed atmosphere, see a bird in flight and marvel at it, put other people at ease or play with pebbles on the beach... Any gesture or act that takes us beyond ourselves and opens our physical and inner eyes to something more than the obvious is done by an artist. Anyone who knows how to live life well is an artist.

If we, as nurses, want to move forward with practice, make our work relevant and have credence in health care, we have to be 'artful'. We have to make it clear that our professional identity is valued and sought after. We have to be different but belong; outrageous but with a purpose; dreaming our dreams but making them applicable.

Anyone who can use ethical principles and theories like an artist, to help us see further, wider and newer perspectives through ethics and morality, needs to be heard and seen. Nurses have always been such artists; therefore they need to be seen and heard. We may need to challenge the tried and tested ways of communicating this, and, for this reason, we have to think in terms of artists because artists look at scenes and colour with fresh eyes.

Ethics is not the dry study of some esoteric subject. When ethics is seen as touching us every day and all day, it becomes lively and colourful. When ethics becomes something that can inspire us and guide us, we are then true artists of society, especially of each other as human beings.

The subjects that I will consider in this chapter are presented with broad brushstrokes. I am not concerned with the details of such thorny questions as pay and conditions, grading structures or even advanced practice. I am not competent to elaborate on these, although I will touch on them indirectly and generally. For many of the ideas put forward in this chapter, I am indebted to Michael Wilson.

Nursing is often described as an art, and people have tried to define what they mean by this. I am not concerned with defining this further but simply with perhaps adding another 'picture' to the art gallery that is nursing. In this way, I hope that some of the ideas developed in earlier chapters will make sense by coming full circle.

Prophets

I was very surprised some years ago, when studying the role of models for ethical decision making (Tschudin, 1995), to come across the idea of prophecy in connection with nursing. Campbell (1986, p. 51) uses the image of 'the fool' as a symbol for those who care for others. Since they do their caring with a lack of self-interest, subjecting themselves to contamination from the ill, hard work, low status and every kind of physical and emotional pain by being around sick and unhealthy people, they must be 'fools'. In this sense, 'fools' are considered to be simpletons and easily exploited. However, Campbell (1986, p. 54) considers that there is also a:

> more active, rumbustious, resilient aspect of the fool... [which] gives a quite different perspective to the nature of folly. It reveals it to be a form of *prophecy*, not in the sense of *fore*telling the future, but in the sense of *forth*telling, of pointing to the signs of the times.

In this capacity, fools challenge the 'accepted norms, conventions and authorities within a society' (p. 55). A clown in a show makes us laugh, but do we laugh at an outsider dressed in fantastic clothes, or do we laugh because something in us is addressed? Who laughs?

Like fools and clowns, nursing must 'seem a little bizarre, a little naïve, and not a little irreverent, in the context of the values which our materialistic culture worships' (Campbell, 1986, p. 59). Perhaps it is that need of having to be cared for, which all of us experience at some time in our lives, that gives us the right to challenge the cultures and ideas, authorities and norms. Perhaps more than many other professionals, nurses know what this means.

Niebuhr (1963, p. 67) makes the point that the prophets of old did not remind their people that they were required to obey a law (deontology) or that they were directed towards as goal (teleology), but, in critical moments, prophets interpreted what was going on. The 'signs of the times' that are to be interpreted vary with cultures, societies and organisations. Campbell (1984, p. 84) speaks of 'the prophetic role of medicine', but the same must also apply to nursing. Professionals, Campbell claims, stand between the weak and the strong in society. They are thus a kind of bridge between patients and clients, and politicians and policy makers. In this position, they are in touch with weakness, vulnerability and disadvantages. They interpret the social context of the weak and therefore need to challenge the social context of the strong. The prophetic voice speaks about this challenge.

Prophecy is not about speculating in the future but of listening to the present and interpreting the 'signs of the times'. It is about *forth*telling it, that is, telling it as it is, speaking about it, making it clear. Prophets need to have a very simple and clear message, and nurses and nursing has one, too: people matter, so their mattering matters; they need to be heard. This means also that nurses matter and their mattering matters; they too need to be heard. The voice that nursing has and needs to find again within itself is today a prophetic one. When nurses make it clear that 'people matter', they speak as prophets as well as realists and compassionate human beings.

Nursing has been aligned with the weak and disadvantaged element in society. Nurses have often allied themselves with patients to the exclusion of challenging the strong, such as governments and rulers. If nursing is to survive, it needs to take on the prophetic role of the challenger much more clearly and readily, otherwise it may lose its voice altogether. The idea that people matter is a strong moral value, and such values 'play a more or less direct role in legitimating or challenging institutional and other social practices' (Jordan and Weedon, 1995, p. 550).

Some of these ideas and theories can be addressed directly. Tornquist (1997, p. 3) states that 'one of the greatest challenges for nurse has been to clarify and define the complex processes which form the art and science of nursing' so that nursing can be reckoned with as an entity. Tornquist's report is a collection of papers from the six regions of the WHO. It is therefore interesting to note that:

> although most nurses would assert that care is a vital component of what nurses do, it is not explicitly mentioned in the papers. (p. 13)

The report points out that, in most of the world, most nurses work in hospitals, 'giving curative and rehabilitative care' (p. 129). While many nurses have a degree of autonomy, many more nurses 'are essentially medical assistants'. Under the heading 'What nurses could do' (p. 130), Tornquist suggests that:

> non-physician primary care providers such as nurses and midwives have been shown to be cost effective. Indeed, studies have found that appropriately prepared nurses can provide as much as 80% of the health care and up to 90% of the paediatric care that is currently delivered by physicians, at equal or better quality and at less cost. Nurses could also be cost effective providers for the world's growing population of elderly.

Clearly, what nurses *do* is important to note. The deeper point, however, is what nurses *are* and what they are willing to be. Gulland (1998b, p. 14) describes the work of a steering group organised by the NHS Confederation and the Institute of Health Services Management. This group:

> has identified four main drivers of change: the development of new technologies and large amounts of information; new power structures in politics, business and community life; the growing importance of our relationship to the environment; and the changing social and cultural world.

The 'ethos of the debate is to make sure that nurses and other health professionals can take ownership of their future' (Gulland, 1998b). The role of the nurse prophets may be to ensure that this happens.

Watson (1987, p. 10) says that Florence Nightingale, in her essay entitled 'Cassandra', wondered why women have passion, intellect and moral activity but not a place in society where these can be exercised. She concludes:

> Like the mythical Cassandra, Nightingale possessed the gift of prophecy and despaired at not being heard. The caring edge of nursing is dedicated to recreating the Cassandra myth by providing places where the passion, intellect, and moral activity of women and nurses can be voiced and heard.

Morality is something very basic in humanity. We learn to be moral just by 'being'. Ethics comes later and has a much more studied aspect to it. We need both, and nursing is about both. Nurses can only be moral 'artists' when they also have ethical understanding. Cassandra always spoke the truth, but nobody would listen. It seems that nurses now need to speak the truth in such a way that they are listened to and heard. They have to speak the truth with passion and intellect. Doing that is the moral activity of women and nurses; this is no doubt also the prophetic activity of nursing.

Leaders

Although I have already touched on the subject of leadership in Chapter 6, I am coming back to it briefly in this setting, considering here the role of the leaders themselves.

Scott (1995, p. 282) writes that:

> in terms of morally sensitive, humane and compassionate practice, one of the most serious failures in nursing and medicine is the general failure within the professions, and among their educators, to identify role models in clinical practice, who would provide students with the ideals of practice that [a] virtuous person provides for students of the virtuous life.

Scott writes from the perspective of Aristotelian virtue ethics, considering that the profession needs to identify 'ethically sensitive role models' (p. 282) for health care practitioners from early in their training:

> If this occurs, the character traits that are being suggested in the literature as being desirable in the health care practitioner may begin to emerge on something more than an ad hoc basis.

According to Aristotle's theory, writes Scott (p. 283), it is important to have 'the appropriate emotions at the appropriate time in a given situation'. She details this in writing that:

> apart from the important issue of the impact of the type, timing and effects of one's emotional reactions on the type of one's character, many of the elements that are seen as important to appropriate, morally praiseworthy practice imply an emotional component (e.g. empathy, sympathy, compassion and care). This means that what one feels is relevant, in the context of health care, to both character and practice.

In a study conducted by Pang and Wong (1998, pp. 424–40) in Hong Kong to elucidate the Chinese practice of 'model emulation', they asked nursing students to describe their experience of positive and negative examples of nursing:

> Positive examples were situations where nurses demonstrated responsible, kind, polite, patient, compassionate and responsive care relevant to patients' needs. Negative examples were situations where nurses were insensitive to patients' feelings, rigid, indifferent, and even hostile to some patients, task oriented, unable to tolerate inefficiency, infringed patients' dignity and privacy, rough in handling patients, and above all, failed to provide responsive care, therefore causing harm to patients.

It may be possible to ask whether nurses who are educated to be kind and respectful in care can be leaders of people, competent at making important decisions, versed in policy making and education and engaging in vision and dialogue about the future of nursing. Can the same people who are skilled at caring intimately for sick and vulnerable people also steer the profession into the future? The answer must be an emphatic 'yes'.

Leaders have to be the people who are able to say the creative 'yes' and 'no' decisively when it matters. They can only do this in relationships, and this they will have learned essentially in their care for people. Truly caring nurses have to inform themselves of all kinds of knowledge, not just that of nursing. Issues of the environment and social, political and spiritual trends and developments have to be the daily learning *milieu* of nurses. Such issues become more urgent in leadership but will have been seen at work and learned in the care of individuals.

The idea that people matter is not restricted to care at a sick person's bedside. The elements of virtuous practice (empathy, sympathy, compassion and care) are also relevant for politicians and managers. The essentials of these elements are listening and responding to the person concerned, which applies to individuals as to society. What matters to the individuals listened to also matters to the wider society. In respecting a suffering person, we respect a suffering society.

Such ideas and questions need to be discussed in classrooms and groups, among colleagues and with clients. The role models in nursing have to be not only good practising nurses, but also leaders of people. They need to foster these qualities in themselves as well as in their students. Nurses need to see and feel that their leaders are people who can be trusted. They are quick to spot deficiencies and are not easily fooled.

To mark the UK's presidency of the European Union, Salvage (1998, pp. 32–3) compiled a report detailing the top nursing jobs in the EU countries. She showed that the UK was leading the EU countries by having the largest Ministry of Health nursing unit (only four other countries even have such units), and having a chief nursing officer in government in each of the UK countries (several countries having either no such posts or only one at advisory level). While this does not guarantee success for nursing, it is encouraging that such posts exist. Nurses in high places do not mean that nursing has good leadership, but it does mean that role models are available. The challenge is that they are and remain credible.

Nursing needs leaders up front, but leadership from the back is just as important. Encouraging, empowering and addressing the potential in a person is perhaps as important for leaders as is the flag waving. Above all, leaders have to be able to listen – to themselves and to their colleagues. Leaders need to be able to judge their own work and role, and their effectiveness in them. They need to know themselves, their strengths and their weaknesses. By affirming that people matter, their leadership of people becomes valid. When they see and hear what matters to people, they will be able to respond in the most appropriate way, according to their talent, role and given power.

Leaders have to be people of vision, and as this is in itself ethical behaviour, we are, as nurses, all called to be leaders. In this sense, we act morally when we fulfil our leadership role.

'Moral artists' are people who dare, who believe in people, who can live with uncertainty, who can be patient and impatient at once, who can speak out and keep still to listen, and who can be both at the front and with those who hurt. Leaders have to be human beings in the fullest sense and not simply puppets or yes-men. Perhaps, in Nightingale's words, they have to be women and men capable of saying the creative 'no' in order to be morally visible. The 'no' here relates to injustice and inequality, as well as to all other practices or forms of repression and abnegation of the principle that people matter.

Sharing

An aspect of the principle that people matter is that there is no division between them and us, those who do and those who are done to, those who care and those who are cared for. There will always be differences in role, but, when we affirm that 'people matter', we are saying that all people matter equally. In nursing, this is of fundamental importance because too often it has not been like that; nurses know this only too well.

> When we take the idea that people matter at face value, everything we do becomes a sharing. When we take ourselves seriously, especially as nurses, we look neither up nor down at other people, but we respect everyone as equal. When we share ourselves, we enable others automatically, which in turn enables us.

A study carried out with older people in continuing care (Ford, 1997, p. 50) showed, among other things, that:

> expert nurses were seen to be knowledgeable, understanding, compassionate and intuitive;
>
> good nurses demonstrate technical competence as well as kindness and compassion;
>
> genuine caring makes a patient feel loved;
>
> being nursed by expert nurses affected the self-esteem of the patients, making them feel valued.

Some of the recommendations made by Ford (1997, p. 50) are that:

> By focusing on older people, research conducted on partnership between patients and nurses may identify useful data on the concept of reciprocity;
>
> studies on the desire for reciprocity by the patient in the nurse–patient relationship may yield useful data;
>
> studies exploring nurses' understanding of the concept of reciprocity may generate useful data for use by nurse educationists;
>
> an investigation into what nurses perceive to be the value of nurses' work with older people may generate further insights into the value of such work;
>
> further research on the nurse–patient relationship and the presence of supportive family networks could further clarify the importance of such relationships.

Some of the patients interviewed wished to establish friendships with their nurses and engage in reciprocal relationships with them. This may particularly be a feature of work with elderly people, who may be more prone to loneliness and increasing isolation, but the same may not be the case in a surgical unit. It is significant, however, that the word 'reciprocity' is mentioned repeatedly in the article, implying that the people interviewed are giving the nurses something. Nurses have perhaps been shy in saying what exactly it is that they are receiving from their patients, apart from the well-known 'job satisfaction'. Noddings (1984, p. 2) makes it clear that rooted in the feminine way of being are 'receptivity, relatedness and responsiveness', and May (1975, p. 33) writes that 'exchange, agreement and reciprocity... mark the professional relationship'. The exchange – the sharing – is therefore something equal, given and taken, and valued by both parties. Clearly, every relationship is different, but what is essentially shared is one's humanity. Patients and clients can hardly share anything else, and, for that matter, nurses cannot *share* anything else either. They can give care and show their expertise, but it is only the human element – the relationship – that can be responded to. By affirming therefore that people matter, we touch again the heart of what life is about and therefore what ethics is about. But dare nurses be friends with their patients? Can patients realistically expect to be friends with nurses? This, I suggest, is what moral artistry is about.

The patterns of diseases and health care are drastically changing in our time. Medicine developed in a time when the population was threatened by infectious diseases such as polio, cholera, plague and tuberculosis. The diseases were controlled as much by environmental factors as by medications. The culture of preventing and attacking disease has, however, remained with us, especially in the idea of isolating people in hospitals when they are ill. It is there that all those associated with cure can be concentrated and can control people and illnesses. What is increasingly clear today is that the pattern of diseases is changing, and hospitals, as we know them today, are becoming obsolete. Today's illnesses are increasingly psychosocial and not amenable to the same ideas of diagnosis–cure. We still think in terms of heart disease, for example, but the reasons for it may not be so much high cholesterol levels as unemployment having led to depression, lack of exercise, an unhealthy diet, meaninglessness and back again in a vicious circle. The cause for the disease is not directly medical but social, political, psychological, environmental and spiritual. The illnesses are interpersonal and intrapersonal first and foremost, and therefore need a different approach to health and disease altogether. Whereas in the past, we concentrated on *cure*, now we need to concentrate on *education* to enable growth through illness. This is largely carried out in the community, at home, in the family and in one's own setting. If much of what we see as 'illness' now is based on a kind of rootlessness, it cannot be cured by uprooting the person even more into special centres of treatment. The sort of care of diseases that we will meet more and more is therefore a care of accompanying a person and befriending in the 'skilled companionship' mode. We need to make a distinction between treating an illness (which will remain a doctor's job) and treating a person (which is a nurse's job). By 'education' I mean not 'teaching' so much as 'leading from', in the true sense of the word: enabling the person to go from the unable to the able and the unknown to the known. Education is also rightly considered increasingly to be a life-long activity and process. This kind of being with others is moral and supportive, and, above all, shows that what matters to people matters.

Indeed, this makes the idea that people matter stronger than ever. The notion of treating the person includes the possibility of referral to a doctor for cure when indicated, but it shows that nursing is the primary contact because nursing contact is more sustained and available. In this paradigm, nurses are not simply dispensers of practical skills but are the educators and enablers who live and work alongside people, fostering, nurturing and caring for people's capacity to live and grow. The emphasis is more strongly on what is right with a person than on what is wrong, bringing nurses more in line with the ideal of the archetype, that is, as being the person who nourishes and strengthens others.

What this points to is a model of nurses as long-term 'companions' – the idea of clinical supervision being similar – to perhaps a number of people. In the UK, we have the models of midwives accompanying a woman through pregnancy and delivery, and health visitors taking over, also on a long-term basis. Just as people are now registered with a GP, they may perhaps one day be 'registered' with a nurse. This relationship, however, may be a much closer one, not simply to be called upon in times of trouble. Such a situation may need to be flexible, inclusive, friendly yet advisory. The relationship would above all demand integrity if it were not to become yet again a relationship based on power. Such relationships have to be learned, sustained and supported. There may need to be elements of give-and-take in the relationships, perhaps even bartering, an idea that is gaining credibility in many local areas.

These ideas may seem rather utopian, but surely the reality is also staring us in the face if we look only a little into the future. It is therefore at this very level that nurses' ethical work is to envision, challenge and run with ideas. It is here that the tenet 'people matter' comes into its own: patients matter and nurses matter. Patients matter because, in this paradigm, they are indeed nurtured and supported, and nurses matter because, in this setting, they are most truly fulfilling their role. At this level, they are sharing: truly sharing themselves and their best skills.

Inclusiveness

The voice of nursing will only be heard when it is an inclusive voice, included in society and including people everywhere.

Nurses do many different tasks the world over, but everywhere they are concerned with people and with their needs. The saying goes that a butterfly flapping its wings over Tokyo affects the weather in London, and, similarly, one can say that a nurse in Lensk, Siberia, affects the care of nurses in the Falkland Islands. This can be a daunting idea but also hugely stimulating, making us aware of the tremendous responsibility we have towards each other. If the voice of nurses and nursing is to be heard, we need to take such ideas much more seriously. The need to learn from each other, locally, nationally and internationally, and work in partnerships is not just novel but a necessity.

As long as nurses insist that they care, they are in danger of excluding themselves. Many people and professions care (my local waste disposal company is called WasteCare) and, in nursing, care can be patronising. If the idea of caring is used to enhance power, there is an enormous danger of its being abused. If nurses use care as their distinguishing feature, their voice will not be heard because people generally will not see this as being relevant to them all of the time. When nurses say loud and clear that 'people matter', people generally will feel themselves to be heard, addressed and included. This means that nurses then have the voice *of* the people and can be a voice *for* the people. It is not *the* voice, because everyone has

a voice when they have been empowered by the support necessary, but it is *a* voice that matters. Such a voice can be specific
in specific situations. The role of advocacy therefore comes
into its own. What matters to individuals, groups and societies
matters also to those who care for or share with them. The
possibility then exists that in some circumstances, nurses speak
for certain people, and in others, people speak for nurses.
This is surely happening anyway, but the possibility that it will
become a more equal undertaking is evident.

This may be more visionary than reality. In Chapter 6, I
argued that to take a visionary stance is an ethical stance because
today's world needs vision to get it out of the morass into which
it has run. In an ideal society, nobody would need to speak on
behalf of others because everyone would have what they needed.
This too may be speculation, although it has been tried. People
and communities – such as the Amish or the Hutterite Brothers
in North America – who ensure that everyone has what they
need and all decisions are made in common, tend to be exclu-
sivists. Beeching (1997, p. 212) says that:

> if your ethical code is based on fleeing evil, you are in a poor posi-
> tion to deal with mammon. Unhappily, also, you enter these frays
> at your peril. Given half a chance, the world will simply kill you.

We can be pure and good with a few other people, but, as
soon as we encounter others, such systems fall because they
have no way of being ethical within a wider context. To be
inclusive means also to be ethical, and surely in the global village
of today, we have no other possibility.

Many examples of inclusive practice are coming to light. The
lead given in such practices by the hospices is remarkable. In
the UK, hospices are now a well-established fact, and many
other countries have copied the idea. There are examples of
experimental GP practices and health centres, and the increasing
number of nursing development units in the UK is encouraging. Primary care groups are envisaged by the government
as part of the 'third way', affirming that the 'needs of patients'
are the starting point (Department of Health, 1998). When people
with vision and passion can say the creative 'no' (or 'enough is
enough'), they then find the necessary energy to change rigid
structures and mind-sets.

Most of these ideas demand indeed a paradigm in which nurses and all health care professionals are much more part of the daily life of all people. If the main emphasis is education rather than cure, everyone has to learn this new language. It may need to start with our state schools. At present, there is a trend of business and industry being involved with schools, and this points indeed to inclusiveness and integration. On the other hand, businesses and industry are interested in having people fit to do jobs when they leave school. This may be too narrow a view. Undoubtedly, workers in every sector of business and industry have to be flexible and multiskilled, able to do several jobs, but the emphasis is still on the doing. We should not forget that we are human *beings* rather than human *doings*. With emphasis on production and skills, we neglect the emphasis on the being and feeling aspect of living. When we stress too much the articulation of logic, we neglect the whole area of living, which most people find to their cost is underdeveloped in later life. The crisis that this causes is then picked up by doctors, counsellors and firms through their pension funds when people retire early because of burnout and breakdown.

The need to be inclusive in living stretches from birth to death, the need for education from school to retirement. If nurses would and could take on the role of 'skilled companion', this would make nursing at once legitimate and vital. While we now still too often shy away from being involved, in this scenario involvement is the bedrock. We would need to think completely differently about relationships. The future looks more person centred than task or cure centred. Nurses in particular would have a central role in education for health and lifestyle. This is a far wider vision than simply 'health promotion' as presently understood. Nurses of the future, are, above all, community builders, the ideas of community also being necessarily redefined. In such communities, the real artists are those who can maintain the community, and nurses are ideally suited to this work.

In such communities, it is the person who counts: people matter more than anything else. The lifestyles of such communities will necessarily vary, but certain things will be common to all. In particular, the skilled companion nurse would be well placed to sustain personalities by nurturing people's individual strengths above all. With strengths affirmed, people will be more at ease with themselves and their environment and possibly be less aggressive and destructive because they are affirmed and empowered rather than feeling the burden of inadequacy and exclusion. Nurses may need to understand illness not just in terms of diagnosis but more like the complementary and alternative therapists do at present, as a manifestation of the imbalance of various forces. These therapies and systems, I believe, will become much more mainstream and integral to all health care, and nurses will therefore need to have a good working knowledge of all forms of healing and caring. They will be able to perform many such tasks themselves or be able to refer to the most appropriate agency.

All kinds of boundaries on maps, not only those within the European Union, are disappearing. With increasing travel, people are much more familiar with other cultures and societies. Communication via the Internet makes global boundaries and physical restrictions of mail services all but obsolete. The boundaries between them and us, professionals and lay, sick and healthy, institutions and individuals, also become blurred. We need to be able to work across boundaries, recognising that much of what we do and are has fuzzy and growing edges. It is at the edges that growth happens more radically than at the centre, where traditions are established. Nurses need to be always at the edges, looking outwards and inwards to possibilities and developments.

Such ideas and visions encourage us to be much more daring with innovations of all kinds. When we think of possibilities of sharing and integration, we have also to consider other ways of living with each other. We may need to think less in terms of opposites and duality, especially in the areas of experience. For many people, the tried and tested certainties and beliefs are no longer applicable or relevant. What they know is their experience, and that may not always be easily explained or accepted. If we can live more socially again, in communities that are accepting of people, such places may also be the centres where 'mattering matters' is considered and reconsidered in a supportive way. Such work necessarily leads far into the realms of the unknown and what may today be termed 'dangerous'.

In Chapter 5, I considered the idea that we need to become more familiar with pain and death and see them less as enemies and more like 'brothers' and 'sisters' again. It may be possible to envisage such communities as places where people live their illness and death positively. In communities, the issues of scarce resources can be more ethically addressed than they can nationally. When people can contribute to and decide their own destinies, perhaps developed over a long time in discussion with a skilled companion, these issues may lose their dread and the drastic decisions that sometimes have to be taken today, thus enriching the whole community.

Our Western psyche concentrates heavily on retributive justice, finding fault and paying for it. It has been said that, in Western churches, a sinner is taken to a court of justice, whereas in the Eastern orthodox church, a sinner is taken to hospital. The emphasis is less on guilt and punishment than on a recognition of falling short of the ideal, needing 'care' rather than 'cure'. Such recognition of falling short of an ideal enables us to look at the ideal and the reason for falling short in a constructive way. The idea of the skilled companion, educator or befriender is also the appropriate symbol here. Together, it may be possible to consider what is happening. Together, we may be able to befriend the chaos, darkness, pain and perhaps the emptiness. A person's experience of these places and states of being can be very frightening, and the person can all too quickly be labelled as psychotic. In such situations, we may be able to see such experiences as helpful for human growth. When people are willing to be skilled companions, they may be able to accompany a person into such dark places without fear, knowing that there is support available always and that such 'journeys' into the human hinterland are necessary for the growth of individuals and societies. Such journeys are clearly not for the faint-hearted, and not everyone may be called upon to accompany others into such depths. The skilled companion may be the advanced practitioner in today's language, but with one difference: the skilled companion is more broadly skilled in human relationships and community building than is perhaps the case today. Many of these ideas may be too idealistic ever to work in reality; many may be too ambitious. My experience is, however, that unless we look for the sky, we will never get past our own myopia.

What I have presented in this book is a vision of an inclusiveness that would place nurses at the very centre of society. As nurses, we have to strive for this position because we have something very good to offer society: we can make the idea that 'people matter' a reality. We do it all the time but at present hampered by tradition, fear and a lack of conviction that has so far inhibited and disabled us. In this last chapter, I have been speculative and imaginary for the sole purpose of highlighting some of the areas in which nurses may be moral artists. My own talents with a paintbrush are limited. I see myself more as the person with the highlighter, pointing to other people's and thinkers' work, pointing to what may be useful in nursing and for nurses and perhaps writing it in such a fashion that it can be considered to be possible. The moral aspect for all of us lies in the willingness to affirm that people matter, that what matters to them matters, and that what is so often given – the pain, illness, darkness and loneliness – has to be pondered, considered, befriended and worked with for it to be of any use. When we include all these facets into our daily life, we become fully human. When we do this, we may feel like the man in the story I recounted in Chapter 2, whose therapist looked at him and 'with love in his eyes said, "I'd like to see you again"'.

This kind of relating and addressing the person, instead of a diagnosis or problem, is crucial for nursing. It is this, rather than any definition, which will take nursing forward and make it legitimate. Underlying this way of being and doing is the conviction and working model that 'people matter'. This will give nursing a professional identity more surely than any label will. How such an identity will evolve and be used depends on every person and on his and her own way of 'mattering'. An identity is not formed overnight but grows and develops.

I hope that these thoughts and ideas can contribute to the debate. Only when the creative 'no' and 'yes' can be used, visions fostered, political points made and support again found at the heart of the experience of work can we be secure enough to push the boundaries out. Humanity and the planet in total demand of us nothing less than visionary artistry.

Bibliography

Affara, F.A. and Styles, M.M. (1993) *Nursing Regulation Guidebook: From Principle to Power*. Geneva: International Council of Nurses.

Albrecht, T.L. (1982) 'What job stress means for the staff nurse', *Nursing Administration Quarterly*, **7**(1): 1–11.

Anderson (1991) Quoted in the National Association for Staff Support publication, 'The Costs of Stress and the Costs and Benefits of Stress Management'.

Andrews, M., Gidman, J. and Humphreys, A. (1998) 'Reflection: does it enhance professional nursing practice?', *British Journal of Nursing*, **7**(7): 413–17.

Anonymous (1993) 'Reaching out', *Nursing Times*, **89**(1): 42.

Anonymous (1998a) 'What would you do?', *Nursing Times*, **94**(2): 34–5.

Anonymous (1998b) 'No way out', *Nursing Standard*, **12**(16): 19.

Antrobus, S. (1998) 'Thoroughly modern leaders', *Nursing Times*, **94**(18): 66–7.

Åström G., Jansson, L., Norberg, A. and Hallberg, I.R. (1993) 'Experienced nurses' narratives of their being in ethically difficult care situations', *Cancer Nursing*, **16**(3): 179–87.

Australian Nursing Council (1993) *Code of Ethics for Nurses in Australia*. Canberra: Australian Nursing Council.

Bagnall, P. (1997) 'Jill of all trades?', *Nursing Times*, **93**(10): 24–6.

Beauchamp, T.L. and Childress, J.F. (1989) *Principles of Biomedical Ethics*, 3rd edn. Oxford: Oxford University Press.

Beeching, P.Q. (1997) *Awkward Reverence*. London: SCM Press.

Benhabib, S. (1992) *Situating the Self; Gender, Community and Postmodernism in Contemporary Ethics*. Cambridge: Polity Press.

Bickley, J. (1997) 'The limits of language: ethical aspects of strike action from a New Zealand perspective', *Nursing Ethics*, **4**(4): 303–12.

Bishop, V. (1998) 'Clinical supervision: what's going on? Results of a questionnaire', *Nursing Times*, **94**(18): 50–3.

Blair, T. (1996) *New Britain; My Vision of a Young Country*. London: Fourth Estate.

Bradshaw, A. (1994) *Lighting the Lamp; The Spiritual Dimension of Nursing Care*. London: Scutari Press.

Briody, M.E. (1996) 'The future of the clinical specialist in the USA', *International Nursing Review*, **43**(1): 17–20, 21–32.

Bruce, L. (1999) 'Religious and spiritual issues in Tschudin, V. (ed.) *Counselling and Older People: An Introductory Guide*. London: Age Concern Books.

Buber, M. (1937) (translated by Smith, R.G., latest impression 1996) *I and Thou*. Edinburgh: T. & T. Clark.

Buchan, J. (1991) *Nurses' Work and Worth: Pay, Careers and Working Patterns of Qualified Nurses* (IMS Report 213). Falmer: Institute of Manpower Studies.

Burrows, R. (1997) 'Carmel: a stark encounter with the human condition', *The Way*, suppl. 89, pp. 97–105.

Butler, P. (1998) 'Robo-nurse on the march', *Nursing Times*, **94**(2): 15–16.

Cain, P. (1997) 'Using clients', *Nursing Ethics*, **4**(6): 465–71.

Callahan, D. (1994) 'Bioethics: private choice and common good', *Hastings Center Report*, **24**(3): 28–31.

Campbell, A.V. (1984) *Moderated love: A Theology of Professional Care*. London: SPCK.

Campbell, A.V. (1986) *Rediscovering Pastoral Care*. London: Darton, Longman & Todd.

Campbell, A.V. (1997) 'Individual' in Boyd, K.M., Higgs, R. and Pinching, A.J. (eds) *The New Dictionary of Medical Ethics*. London: BMJ Publishing.

Campbell, C.S. (1993) 'Gridlock on the Oregon Trail', *Hastings Center Report*, **23**(4): 6–7.

Carlisle, D. (1994) 'Plane speaking', *Nursing Times*, **90**(38): 14–15.

Carlisle, D. (1997) 'Why are we losing all our experienced nurses?', *Nursing Times*, **93**(13): 26–9.

Carlisle, D. (1998) 'Front line battle for human rights', *Nursing Times*, **94**(21): 40–1.

Cassell, E.J. (1993) 'The Sorcerer's broom: medicine's rampant technology', *Hastings Center Report*, **23**(6): 32–9.

Castledine, G. (1997a) 'What is happening to morale in nursing?', *British Journal of Nursing*, **6**(13): 773.

Castledine, G. (1997b) 'Political awareness in nursing in 1997', *British Journal of Nursing*, **6**(1): 58.

Castledine, G. (1998) 'Link between the arts and the experience of nursing', *British Journal of Nursing*, **7**(8): 493.

Cavill, G. (1998) Letter, *Nursing Times*, **94**(5): 22.

Chambers, R. (1998) *Clinical Effectiveness Made Easy; First Thoughts on Clinical Governance*. Abingdon: Radcliffe Medical Press.

Chambliss, D.F. (1996) *Beyond Caring; Hospitals, Nurses, and the Social Organization of Ethics*. Chicago: University of Chicago Press.

Cheek, J. and Rudge, T. (1995) 'Only connect... feminism and nursing', pp. 315–32, in Gray, G. and Pratt, R. (eds) *Scholarship in the Discipline of Nursing*. Melbourne: Churchill Livingstone.

Chinombo, A.M. (1998) 'Empowering communities – a strategy used in Malawi', *International Nursing Review*, **45**(3): 81–4, 88.

Churchill, L.R. (1994) 'Rejecting principlism, affirming principles', pp. 321–31 in DuBose, E.R., Hamel, R. and O'Connell, L.J. (eds) *A Matter of Principles? Ferment in U.S. Bioethics.* Valley Forge, PA: Trinity Press.

Collière, M.F. (1986) 'Invisible care and invisible women as health care providers', *International Journal of Nursing Studies*, **23**(2): 95–112.

Confederation of British Industry (1987) Quoted in the National Association for Staff Support publication, 'The Costs of Stress and the Costs and Benefits of Stress Management'.

Crawford, J., Kippax, S., Onyx, J., Gault, U. and Benton, P. (1992) *Emotion and Gender; Constructing Meaning from Memory.* London: Sage.

Cutliffe, J.R., Epling, M., Cassedy, P., McGregor, J., Plant, N. and Butterworth, T. (1998) 'Ethical dilemmas in clinical supervision. 1: Need for guidelines', *British Journal of Nursing*, **7**(15): 920–3.

Damasio, A.R. (1994) *Descartes' Error: Emotion, Reason, and the Human Brain.* New York: Grosset/Putman.

David, A. and Hopkins, S. (1998) 'Model partnerships', *Nursing Times*, **94**(23): 38–40.

Davies, C. (1996a) 'Cloaked in a tattered illusion', *Nursing Times*, **92**(45): 44–6.

Davies, C. (1996b) 'A new vision of professionalism', *Nursing Times*, **92**(46): 54–6.

Denner, S. (1995) 'Extending professional practice: benefits and pitfalls', *Nursing Times*, **91**(14): 27–9.

Dennett, D.C. (1984) 'Computer models and the mind – a view from the east pole', *Times Literary Supplement*, December. In Zohar, D. (1991) *The Quantum Self.* London: Flamingo.

Department of Health (1994) *The Challenges for Nursing and Midwifery in the 21st Century* (The Heathrow Debate). London: Department of Health.

Department of Health (1998) *The New NHS, Modern, Dependable* (Cm 3807). London: Department of Health.

Dimond, B. (1998) 'Legal aspects of clinical supervision. 1: Employer vs employee', *British Journal of Nursing*, **7**(7): 393–5.

Dobb, J. and Small, M. (1997) Crying together, laughing together, *Nursing Times*, **93**(31): 36–7.

Durgahee, T. (1997) 'Reflective practice: nursing ethics through story telling', *Nursing Ethics*, **4**(2): 135–46.

El-Bakkali-Bellini, F. (1997) 'Spiritualité: la quatrième dimension des soins', *Krankenpflege/Soins infirmiers*, **7**: 54–8.

Evans, L. (1997) 'The emotional costs', (letter), *Nursing Times*, **93**(30): 22.

Fairbairn, G. and Mead, D. (1990) 'Therapeutic storytelling', *Paediatric Nursing*, **2**(6): 11–12.

Farrington, A. (1997) 'Strategies for reducing stress and burnout in nursing', *British Journal of Nursing*, **6**(1): 44–9.

Farrington, A. and Geoghegan, J. (1995) 'Shared governance: an approach to empowering nurses', *British Journal of Nursing*, **4**(13): 734–5.

Faulder, C. (1985) *Whose Body Is It? The Troubling Issue of Informed Consent*. London: Virago.

Fielding, P. and Woan, M. (1998) 'In sickness and in health', *Nursing Times*, **94**(7): 36–7.

Finnis, J. (1980) *Natural Law and Natural Rights*. Oxford: Clarendon Press.

Flatt, S. (1997) 'The issue we must all tackle' (letter), *Nursing Times*, **93**(3): 24.

Ford, P. (1997) 'Older people's views of continuing care', *Nursing Times*, **93**(14): 50–1.

Fowler, J. (1996) 'Clinical supervision: what do you do after saying hello?', *British Journal of Nursing*, **5**(6): 382–5.

Frankl, V.E. (1962) *Man's Search for Meaning; An Introduction to Logotherapy*. London: Hodder & Stoughton.

Galbally, R. (1996) 'Sharing wisdom and responsibility – a view from Australia', *World Health Forum*, **17**(4): 340–2.

Gallagher, U. (1995) 'Medical and nursing ethics: never the twain?', *Nursing Ethics*, **2**(2): 95–102.

Garbett, R. (1997) 'Organising for the future', *Nursing Times*, **93**(17): 40–1.

Garbett, R. (1998) 'It's tough at the top', *Nursing Times*, **94**(18): 68–9.

Giddens, A. (1997) *Sociology*, 3rd edn. Cambridge: Polity Press.

Gilligan, C. (1982) *In a Different Voice; Psychological Theory and Women's Development*. Cambridge, MA: Harvard University Press.

Gillon, R. (1986) *Philosophical Medical Ethics*. Chichester: Wiley.

Glover, D. (1998) 'A chance to make your mark', *Nursing Times*, **94**(19): 17.

Gordon, R. (undated) *The Location of Archetypal Experience* (Pamphlet 212). London: Guild of Pastoral Psychology.

Goudzwaard, B. and de Lange, H. (1995) *Beyond Poverty and Affluence; Toward an Economy of Care* (translated by Vander Vennen, M.R.). Geneva: WCC Publications.

Gough, P. (1998) 'The future is yours', *Nursing Times*, **94**(26): 30–2.

Griffiths, P. (1997) 'In search of the pioneers of nurse-led care', *Nursing Times*, **93**(21): 46–8

Grove-White, R. (1995) 'Top-down solutions', *Resurgence*, **172**: 22–4.

Gulland, A. (1998a) 'Revving up for life in the pilot seat', *Nursing Times*, **94**(1): 14–15

Gulland, A. (1998b) 'A 2020 vision of the future', *Nursing Times*, **94**(25): 14.

Gulland, A. and Payne, D. (1997) 'Daisy chain power', *Nursing Times*, **93**(34): 14–15.

Hancock, C. (1998) 'The long and winding road', *Nursing Times*, **94**(2): 24.

Handy, C. (1997) *The Hungry Spirit: Beyond Capitalism, a Quest for Purpose in the Modern World*. London: Hutchinson.

Harris, T.A. (1973) *I'm OK – You're OK*. London: Pan.

Harwood, A. (1997) 'What kind of leader are you?', *Nursing Times*, **93**(12): 66–9.

Hastings Center (1998) 'Case study: an alert and incompetent self; the irrelevance of advance directives', *Hastings Center Report*, **28**(1): 28.

Heslop, L. and Oates, J. (1995) 'The discursive formation of caring', pp. 259–80 in Gray, G. and Pratt, R. (eds) *Scholarship in the Discipline of Nursing*. Melbourne: Churchill Livingstone.

Hoda, S. (1995) 'Gandhi's talisman', *Resurgence*, **172**: 10–13.

Huey, F.L. (1988) 'How nurses would change U.S. health care'. *American Journal of Nursing 88*: 1482–93, in Watson, J. (1993) *Advanced Nursing Practice and What Might Be*. Based upon a paper delivered at Third National Clinical Nurse Specialist Conference, 'Caring in advanced practice: ethical challenges, knowledge development, innovative strategies', Ottawa, Ontario.

Hunt, G. (1995) 'Introduction: Whistleblowing and the breakdown of accountability', pp xiii–xxix, and 'Conclusion: A new accountability?', pp. 154–64 in Hunt, G. (ed.) *Whistleblowing in the Health Service; Accountability, Law and Professional Practice*. London: Edward Arnold.

Hunt, G. (1996) 'Some ethical ground rules for BSE and other public health threats', *Nursing Ethics*, **3**(3): 263–7.

Illich, I. (1976) *Limits to Medicine; Medical Nemesis: The Expropriation of Health*. Harmondsworth: Penguin.

International Council of Nurses (1972) *Code for Nurses*. Geneva: International Council of Nurses.

International Council of Nurses (1997) 'ICN plans for nursing's future directions. *News*, **11**(January) (ICN/97/3).

Irvine, M. (1995) 'Thoughts and meditations on the base chakra', *Radionic Journal*, **41**(1): 15–22.

Jacobs, M. (1996) *The Politics of the Real World* (written and edited for the Real World Coalition). London: Earthscan Publications.

Jenkins, D. (1966) *The Glory of Man*. London: SCM Press.

Johnson, R.A. (1977) *She: Understanding Feminine Psychology*. New York: Harper & Row.

Johnstone, M.J. (1998) 'Advancing nursing ethics: time to set a new global agenda?', *International Nursing Review*, **45**(2): 43.

Jordan, G. and Weedon, C. (1995) *Cultural Politics: Class, Gender, Race and the Postmodern World.* Oxford: Blackwell.

Joseph Rowntree Foundation (1997) Changing mortality ratios in local areas of Britain 1950s–1990s, *Social Policy Research*, **126**.

Jowett, S. (1997) 'The impact of new scope', *Nursing Times*, **93**(52): 36–7.

Jung, C.G. (1964) *Man and his Symbols.* London: Pan Books.

Katsuragi, S. (1997) 'Better working conditions won by "Nurse Wave" action: Japanese nurses' experience of getting a new law by their militant campaign', *Nursing Ethics*, **4**(4): 313–22.

Kenny, C. (1997) 'Nurses the key to health savings', *Nursing Times*, **93**(34): 7.

Kenny, C. (1998) 'Nurse MPs "out of touch"', *Nursing Times*, **94**(19): 12.

Kocher, B. (1997) 'Analyser, mais sans étouffer l'humain', *Krankenpflege/Soins infirmiers*, **6**: 56–64.

Kuhse, H. (1997) *Caring: Nurses, Women and Ethics.* Oxford: Blackwell.

Laishley, F.J. (1998) 'Doing the truth in love', *The Way*, suppl. 91: 112–22.

Langstaff, D. and Gray, B. (1997) 'Flexible roles: a new model in nursing practice', *British Journal of Nursing*, **6**(11): 635–8.

Lawler, J. (1991) *Behind the Screens; Nursing, Somology, and the Problem of the Body.* Melbourne: Churchill Livingstone.

Leners, D. and Beardslee, N.Q. (1997) 'Suffering and ethical caring: incompatible entities', *Nursing Ethics*, **4**(5): 361–9.

Linzey, A. (1997) 'Ethical and theological objections to animal cloning', *Bulletin of Medical Ethics*, **131**: 18–22.

Lowry, M. (1998) 'Clinical supervision for the development of nursing practice', *British Journal of Nursing*, **7**(9): 553–4, 556–7.

Macara, S. (1996) Response in Davies, C. 'A cloak to fit all?', *Nursing Times*, **92**(47): 44–6.

Macara, S. (1997) 'Professionalism' in Boyd, K.M., Higgs, R. and Pinching, A.J. (1997) *The New Dictionary of Medical Ethics.* London: BMJ Publishing.

McTaggart, L. (1998) 'Cheaper options to lower cholesterol', *What Doctors Don't Tell You*, **9**(2): 9.

Macy, J. (1998) 'The great turning', *Resurgence*, **186**(Jan/Feb): 28–9.

Marks-Maran, D. (1997) 'Intuition: "just knowing" in nursing', pp. 92–108 in Marks-Maran, D. and Rose, P. (eds) *Reconstructing Nursing: Beyond Art and Science.* London: Baillière Tindall.

May, W.F. (1975) 'Code, covenant, contract, or philanthropy', *Hastings Center Report*, **5**: 29–38.

Mazhindu, D. (1998) 'Emotional healing', *Nursing Times*, **94**(6): 26–8.

Meadows, D. (1995) 'Seven Blunders', *Resurgence*, **172**: 13.

Mordacci, R. and Sobel, R. (1998) 'Health: a comprehensive concept', *Hastings Center Report*, **28**(1): 34–7.

Morrison, P. and Burnard, P. (1997) *Caring and Communicating; The Interpersonal Relationship in Nursing*, 2nd edn. Basingstoke: Macmillan.

Morrissey, M.V. (1997) 'Extending the theory of awareness contexts by examining the ethical issues faced by nurses in terminal care', *Nursing Ethics*, **4**(5): 370–9.

Mort, L. (1996) 'Critical of care', *Nursing Times*, **92**(19): 40–1.

Murray, C. (1998) 'Nurses may end up being jacks of all trades', *British Journal of Nursing*, **7**(2): 65.

National Association for Staff Support (1992a) *The Costs of Stress and the Costs and Benefits of Stress Management*. Woking: National Association for Staff Support.

National Association for Staff Support (1992b) *A Charter for Staff Support*. Woking: National Association for Staff Support.

Navone, J. (1977) *Towards a Theology of Story*. Slough: St Paul Publications.

New Internationalist (1998) Letters page, (298): 5.

Niebuhr, H.R. (1963) *The Responsible Self*. New York: Harper & Row.

Noddings, N. (1984) *Caring: A Feminine Approach to Ethics and Moral Education*. Berkeley, CA: University of California Press.

Nolan, M. (1996) 'Is nursing becoming a disembodied profession?', *British Journal of Nursing*, **5**(17): 1030.

Norberg, A., Udén, G. (1995) 'Gender differences in moral reasoning among physicians, registered nurses and enrolled nurses engaged in geriatric and surgical care', *Nursing Ethics*, **2**(3): 233–42.

Nortvedt, P. (1998) 'Sensitive judgement: an inquiry into the foundations of nursing ethics', *Nursing Ethics*, **5**(5): 385–92.

Nuffield Trust (1998) *Improving the Health of the NHS Workforce*. Report of the partnership on the health of the NHS workforce, written by Williams, S., Michie, S., and Pattani, S. London: Nuffield Trust.

Nyberg, J. (1994) 'Implementing Watson's theory of caring' in Watson, J. (ed.) *Applying the Art and Science of Human Caring*. New York: National League for Nursing Press.

O'Connor, T. (1994) 'Strikes gain political favour', *Nursing New Zealand*, **1**: 16–17.

Oppenheimer, H. (1988) *Looking Before and After*. London: Fount Paperbacks.

Oppenheimer, H. (1992) 'Abortion: a sketch for a Christian view', *Studies in Christian Ethics*, **5**(2): 46–60.

Oppenheimer, H. (1995) 'Mattering', *Studies in Christian Ethics*, **8**(1): 60–76.

Oulton, J. (1996) 'Human resources are the key – the nurses' view', *World Health Forum*, **17**(4): 343–4.

Oxford Dictionary of Quotations (1993) (4th edn) Partington, A. (ed.) London: Quality Paperbacks direct by arrangement with OUP.

Pang, M.S. and Wong, K.T. (1998) 'Cultivating a moral sense of nursing through model emulation', *Nursing Ethics*, **5**(5): 424–40.

Parker, R.S. (1990) 'Nurses' stories: The search for a relational ethic of care', *Advances in Nursing Science*, **13**(1): 31–40.

Pattison, S. (1997) *The Faith of the Managers: When Management Becomes Religion*. London: Cassell.

Paul, H. (1998) 'Colonization of life', *Resurgence*, **188**: 14–15.

Positive News (1997) 'In brief'; **12**: 3 (col. 5).

Proctor, B. (undated) 'Supervision: a cooperative exercise in account-ability', pp. 21–34 in Marken, M. and Payne, M. (eds) *Enabling and Ensuring*. Leicester: National Youth Bureau and Council for Education and Training in Youth and Community Work.

Puls, J. (1993) *Seek Treasures in Small Fields*. London: Darton, Longman & Todd.

Quick, R. (1997) 'A health care revolution', *Nursing Times*, **93**(29): 17.

Rabbin, R. (1998) 'Seeking truth', *Resurgence*, **188**: 23.

Rachlis, M. and Kushner, C. (1989) 'Second Opinion: What's wrong with Canada's health care system and how to fix it'. Toronto, Ont.: HarperCollins. In Watson, J. (1993) 'Advanced nursing practice and what might be'. Based upon a paper presented at the Third National Clinical Nurse Specialist Conference 'Caring in advanced practice: ethical challenges, knowledge development, innovative strategies', Ottawa, Ontario.

Radford Ruether, R. (1983) *Sexism and God-talk*. London: SCM Press.

De Raeve, L. (1998) 'Maintaining integrity through clinical supervision', *Nursing Ethics*, **5**(6): 489–95.

Reason, P. (1998) 'A participatory world', *Resurgence*, **186**: 42–4.

Reiser, S.J. (1994) 'The ethical life of health care organizations', *Hastings Center Report*, **24**(6): 28–35.

Rickard, M., Kuhse, H. and Singer, P. (1996) 'Caring and justice: a study of two approaches to health care ethics', *Nursing Ethics*, **3**(2): 212–23.

Roach, M.S. (1984) *Caring: The Human Mode of Being, Implications for Nursing*. Toronto: University of Toronto.

Roach, M.S. (1992) *The Human Act of Caring; A Blueprint for the Health Professions*, revised edn. Ottawa: Canadian Hospital Association Press.

Roberts, K. (1995) 'Theoretical, clinical and research scholarship: connections and distinctions', pp. 211–26 in Gray, G. and Pratt, R. (eds) *Scholarship in the Discipline of Nursing*. Melbourne: Churchill Livingstone.

Rogers, C.R. (1980) *A Way of Being*. Boston: Houghton Mifflin.

Rolfe, G. (1996) *Closing the Theory–Practice Gap*. Oxford: Butterworth Heinemann.

Roszak, T. (1995) *The Making of a Counter Culture*. London: University of California Press.

Routasalo, P. (1997) 'Touch in the nursing care of elderly patients', Doctoral Dissertation, University of Turku, Finland.

Rowden, R. (1998) 'Vile bodies', *Nursing Times*, **94**(18): 24.

Royal College of Nursing (1991) Quoted in the National Association for Staff Support publication, 'The Costs of Stress and the Costs and Benefits of Stress Management'.

Royal College of Nursing (1996) *Developing Leaders; A Guide to Good Practice*. London: Royal College of Nursing.

Salvage, J. (1997) 'Journey to the centre', *Nursing Times*, **93**(17): 28–9.

Salvage, J. (1998) 'Taking the lead', *Nursing Times*, **94**(18): 32–3.

Sams, D. (1998) 'When knowledge is power', *Nursing Times*, **94**(5): 77–9.

Scott, H. (1996) 'Unwanted medicine: the delegation of doctors' roles', *British Journal of Nursing*, **5**(17): 1028.

Scott, H. (1998) 'Government nursing initiatives are not enough', *British Journal of Nursing*, **7**(9): 508.

Scott, P.A. (1995) 'Aristotle, nursing and health care ethics', *Nursing Ethics*, **2**(4): 279–85.

Secretary of State for Health (1997) *The New NHS*. London: Stationery Office.

Secretary of State for Health (1998) *Our Healthier Nation; A Contract for Health*, Cm 3852. London: Stationery Office.

Senge, P.M. (1990) *The Fifth Discipline: The Art and Practice of the Learning Organization*. London: Century Business.

Sheldrake, R. and Fox, M. (1996) *Natural Grace: Dialogues on Science and Spirituality*. London: Bloomsbury.

Shepherdson, J. (1992) 'Being there', *Nursing Times*, **88**(10): 35.

Sidgwick, H. (1907) *The Methods of Ethics*, 7th edn. London: Macmillan.

Skolimowski, H. (1994) *The Participatory Mind*. London: Arkana.

Smith, G. R. (1997) 'Creating community power in health care', *International Nursing Review*, **44**(4): 105–9, 120.

Snee, N. and Salter, B. (1997) 'Old flames, new desires', *Nursing Times*, **93**(30): 40–1.

Sofaer, B. (1994) 'Achieving a better life on the planet. Are we our "brothers'" keepers?', *Nursing Ethics*, **1**(3): 173–7.

Stewart, W. (1992) *An A–Z of Counselling Theory and Practice*. London: Chapman & Hall.

Stoter, D. (1995) *Spiritual Aspects of Health Care*. London: Mosby.

Styles, M.M. (1989) *On Specialisation in Nursing: Toward a New Empowerment*. Kansas City: American Nurses' Foundation.

Summers, S. (1992) 'A long night', *Nursing Times*, **88**(19): 47.

Talento, B. (1995) 'Social policy and health care delivery', pp. 129–70 in Deloughery, G.L. (ed.) *Issues and Trends in Nursing*, 2nd edn. St Louis, MO: Mosby.

Taylor, J.V. (1972) *The Go-Between God*. London: SCM Press.

Thomas, P. (1995) 'A study of the effectiveness of staff support groups', *Nursing Times*, **91**(48): 36–9.

Tornquist, E. (ed.) (1997) *Nursing Practice Around the World*. Geneva: Nursing/Midwifery Health Systems Development Programme, World Health Organization.

Tronto, J.C. (1993) *Moral Boundaries; A Political Argument for an Ethic of Care*. London: Routledge.

Tschudin, V. (1992) *Ethics in Nursing; The Caring Relationship*, 2nd edn. Oxford: Butterworth Heinemann.

Tschudin, V. (1994) *Deciding Ethically; A Practical Approach to Nursing Challenges*. London: Baillière Tindall.

Tschudin,V. (1995) 'The role of models for decision making in an ethic of care in nursing', MA Dissertation, University of East London, London.

Tschudin, V. (1997) 'Nursing as a moral art', pp. 64–90 in Marks-Maran, D. and Rose, P. (eds) *Reconstructing Nursing; Beyond Art and Science*. London: Baillière Tindall.

Türcke, C. (1997) *What Price Religion?* (translated by Bowden J.). London: SCM Press.

UKCC (1992a) *Code of Professional Conduct*. London: United Kingdom Central Council for Nursing, Midwifery and Health Visiting.

UKCC (1992b) *The Scope of Professional Practice*. London: United Kingdom Central Council for Nursing, Midwifery and Health Visiting.

UKCC (1996) *Guidelines for Professional Practice*. London: United Kingdom Central Council for Nursing, Midwifery and Health Visiting.

UKCC (1998a) *Guidelines for Mental Health and Learning Disabilities Nursing*. London: United Kingdom Central Council for Nursing, Midwifery and Health Visiting.

UKCC (1998b) 'UKCC considers record number of misconduct complaints about nurses, midwives and health visitors'. Press statement 37/1998. London: United Kingdom Central Council for Nursing, Midwifery and Health Visiting.

US Congress, Office of Technological Assessment (1986) 'Nurse practitioners, physician assistants and certified nurse midwives: a policy analysis' (Health Technology Case Study 37) OTA-HCS-37, p. 5. Washington, DC: US Government Printing Office, in Watson, J. (1993) 'Advanced nursing practice and what might be'. Based upon a paper delivered at Third National Clinical Nurse Specialist Conference, 'Caring in advanced practice: ethical challenges, knowledge development, innovative strategies', Ottawa, Ontario.

Uys, L. (1996) 'Policy options for a regulatory body for nursing in South Africa', *Nursing Ethics*, **3**(4): 345–56.

Vaughan, B. (1996) 'Swiss nurses scrutinize health costs', (news item), *International Nursing Review*, **43**(5): 133–4.

Wall Street Journal (1993) 'Review and Outlook: Nurses' Lib', 13th August. Trenton, NJ: Dow Jones, in Watson, J. (1993) *Advanced Nursing Practice and What Might Be*. Based upon a paper delivered at Third National Clinical Nurse Specialist Conference, 'Caring in advanced practice: ethical challenges, knowledge development, innovative strategies', Ottawa, Ontario.

Walton, K. (1994) Proceedings of the Aristotelian Society, Supplementary volume in Oppenheimer, H. 'Mattering', *Studies in Christian Ethics*, **8**(1): 60–76.

Watson, J. (1987) 'Nursing on the caring edge: metaphorical vignettes', *Advances in Nursing Science*, **10**(1): 10–18.

Watson, J. (1993) *Advanced Nursing Practice and What Might Be*. Based upon a paper delivered at Third National Clinical Nurse Specialist Conference, 'Caring in advanced practice: ethical challenges, knowledge development, innovative strategies', Ottawa, Ontario.

Watson, J. (1994) *Applying the Art and Science of Human Caring*. New York: National League for Nursing Press.

Wells, R. (1998) 'It's good to listen', *Police Ethics*, **1**(April): 5–9.

Wheeler, H.H. (1998) 'Nurse occupational stress research. 5: Sources and determinants of stress', *British Journal of Nursing*, **7**(1): 40–3.

Wilkinson, J. (1998) 'Noncompliance by patients: a response to Professor Dimond', *Nursing Ethics*, **5**(2): 167–72.

Williams, S., Michie, S. and Pattani, S. (1998) *Improving the Health of the NHS Workforce*. (report of the partnership on the health of the NHS workforce). London: Nuffield Trust.

Wilson, J. (1998) 'Incident reporting', *British Journal of Nursing*, **7**(11): 670–1.

Wilson, M. (1976) 'Death and society', pp. 52–71 in Millard, D.W. (ed.) *Religion and Medicine*. London: SCM Press.

Wilson, M. (1993) A response to Birmingham Health Authority's publication, *Towards a Healthy Birmingham*. Paper delivered at a conference organised by BHA.

Wolinsky, S. (1994) *The Tao of Chaos: Essence and the Enneagram*. Connecticut: Bramble.

Wordsworth Dictionary of Biography (1994) Ware: Wordsworth Editions.

Worth, C. (1997) 'Complementary therapies and the NHS: added value?' Printed copy of a presentation given by Worth, C. and Ruddlesden, J. to Parliamentary Group for Complementary and Alternative Medicine at House of Commons, 28 January.

Wright, S. (1997) 'Free the spirit', *Nursing Times*, **93**(17): 30–2.

Index